Principles &
Practice of Nurse
Prescribing

Sara Miller McCune founded SAGE Publishing in 1965 to support the dissemination of usable knowledge and educate a global community. SAGE publishes more than 1000 journals and over 800 new books each year, spanning a wide range of subject areas. Our growing selection of library products includes archives, data, case studies and video. SAGE remains majority owned by our founder and after her lifetime will become owned by a charitable trust that secures the company's continued independence.

Los Angeles | London | New Delhi | Singapore | Washington DC | Melbourne

Principles & Practice of Nurse Prescribing

Jill Gould
Heather Bain

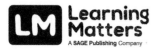

Learning Matters
A SAGE Publishing Company
1 Oliver's Yard
55 City Road
London EC1Y 1SP

SAGE Publications Inc.
2455 Teller Road
Thousand Oaks, California 91320

SAGE Publications India Pvt Ltd
B 1/I 1 Mohan Cooperative Industrial Area
Mathura Road
New Delhi 110 044

SAGE Publications Asia-Pacific Pte Ltd
3 Church Street
#10-04 Samsung Hub
Singapore 049483

Editor: Laura Walmsley
Senior project editor: Chris Marke
Cover design: Wendy Scott
Typeset by: C&M Digitals (P) Ltd, Chennai, India
Printed in the UK

First edition published in 2022

Library of Congress Control Number: 2021947635

British Library Cataloguing in Publication Data

A catalogue record for this book is available from the British Library

ISBN 978-1-5264-6991-5
ISBN 978-1-5264-6990-8 (pbk)

At SAGE we take sustainability seriously. Most of our products are printed in the UK using responsibly sourced papers and boards. When we print overseas we ensure sustainable papers are used as measured by the PREPS grading system. We undertake an annual audit to monitor our sustainability.

Contents

TRANSFORMING NURSING PRACTICE

Transforming Nursing Practice is a series tailor made for pre-registration student nurses. Each book addresses a core topic and is:

 Clearly written and easy to read

 Full of active learning features

 Mapped to the NMC Standards of proficiency for registered nurses

 Focused on applying theory to everyday nursing practice

Each book addresses a core topic and has been carefully developed to be simple to use, quick to read and written in clear language.

An invaluable series of books that explicitly relates to the NMC standards. Each book covers a different topic that students need to explore in order to develop into a qualified nurse... I would recommend this series to all Pre-Registered nursing students whatever their field or year of study.

LINDA ROBSON,
Senior Lecturer at Edge Hill University

Many titles in the series are on our recommended reading list and for good reason - the content is up to date and easy to read. These are the books that actually get used beyond training and into your nursing career.

EMMA LYDON,
Adult Student Nursing

ABOUT THE SERIES EDITORS

DR MOOI STANDING is an Independent Academic Nursing Consultant (UK and international) responsible for the core knowledge, personal and professional learning skills titles. She has invaluable experience as an NMC Quality Assurance Reviewer of educational programmes, and as a Professional Regulator Panellist on the NMC Practice Committee. Mooi is also a Board member of Special Olympics Malaysia.

DR SANDRA WALKER is a Clinical Academic in Mental Health working between North Bristol Trust and Southern Health Trust. She is series editor for the mental health nursing titles. She is a Qualified Mental Health Nurse with a wide range of clinical experience spanning 30 years and spent several years working as a mental health lecturer at Southampton University.

BESTSELLING TEXTBOOKS

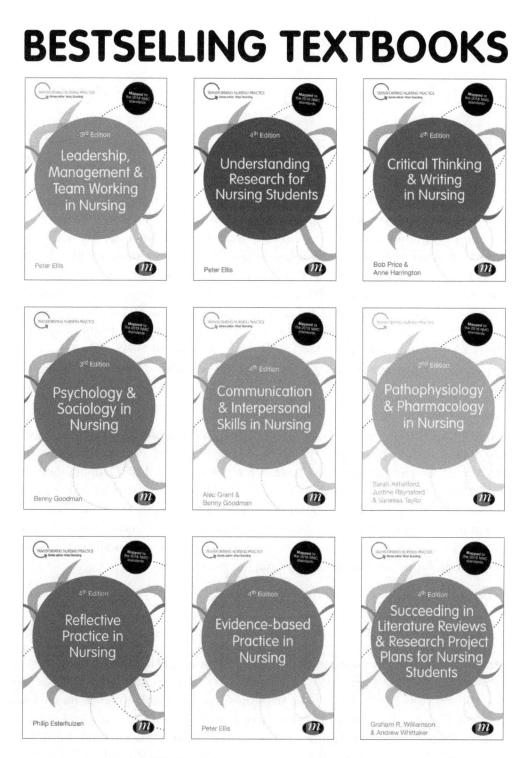

You can find a full list of textbooks in the *Transforming Nursing Practice* series at
uk.sagepub.com/TNP-series

About the authors and contributors

Authors

Dr Heather Bain (EdD, FQNIS, FHEA, PGCert, HELT, BA, DipDN, RGN) is Academic Strategic Lead: Learning, Teaching and Assessment with overall responsibility for all academic programmes and courses within the School of Nursing, Midwifery and Paramedic Practice at Robert Gordon University. Since coming into education in 2002 she has led the implementation of the Extended Nurse Prescribing course and subsequently became the course leader of the post-registration district nurse course and then led the Masters courses and CPD portfolio within the School. Heather has actively promoted community nursing throughout the UK, being a member of the Association of District Nurse and Community Nurse Educators, a Fellow of QNIS and on a number of national working groups. She is also one of the coordinators behind @weDistrictNurse on Twitter.

Jill Gould (MSc PGDip SFHEA, QN, BSc SPQDN, RGN) has been a registered nurse since 1983, a district nurse and prescriber since 1999 and a senior lecturer since 2006. She is currently Programme Leader for the Non-medical (Independent and supplementary) prescribing programmes at the University of Derby, and external examiner for other prescribing programmes. She is a Queen's Nurse, a member of the Association for Prescribers and the Association of District Nurse and Community Nurse Educators. Having spent her formative nursing years in Canada, Jill is an avid supporter of community, district nursing and prescribing by nurses and midwives.

Contributors

Professor Barry Strickland-Hodge (MSc, PhD, FRPharmS, FHEA) is currently Visiting Professor of Prescribing Practice at the University of Leeds and doctoral supervisor at the University of Derby. In 2003 he developed the prescribing course for pharmacists at the University of Leeds. He was appointed Director of the Academic Unit of Pharmacy, Radiography and Healthcare Science in 2012 and Visiting Professor in 2016 both in Leeds. He was designated Fellow of the Royal Pharmaceutical Society in 2008. He has a number of books in information and prescribing, the latest being *Prescribing for Pharmacists* in 2019 and *Practical Prescribing for Medical Students* in 2014.

Alan Bloomer (MPHARM, PG Dip, IP) is a pharmacist with over 17 years' experience working across all sectors of healthcare, including primary and secondary care. He gained his independent prescribing in 2011 and has not looked back, running clinics within general practice and managing patients in acute care. He now works mainly in academia, lecturing across several universities on non-medical prescribing programmes including the universities of Canterbury, Derby and Salford. He enjoys working in clinical practice within secondary care when time permits, especially across Care of the Elderly. In his spare time, you will find him in the hills of the Peak District.

Acknowledgements

The authors would like to acknowledge the work of Ashelford *et al.* in their textbook *Pathophysiology and Pharmacology in Nursing* (2019) and thank them for the use of selected figures.

We would like to thank Jennifer Lee and Rachel Lewis (pharmacist lecturers and independent prescribers, University of Derby) for their valued contributions to the pharmacology chapter, and Tony Daly (Senior Lecturer and independent prescriber, UoD) for his influence throughout in never discussing the 'what' without the 'why'.

Molly Courtenay, author of the first *Nurse Prescribing* textbook, has generously provided a contribution and supported the book from its early days.

A debt of gratitude is owed to Baroness Julia Cumberlege for recognising many years ago in her report into community nursing the ability of nurses to safely and expertly take on the role of prescribers for the betterment of people in their care.

Foreword

During the past two decades there have been significant developments worldwide regarding the extension of nursing roles to include prescribing capability. Many thousands of nurses in the UK can now prescribe medicines and their numbers are steadily rising to fulfil the workforce needs of the NHS. The inclusion of prescribing knowledge and skills now in pre-registration programmes will only facilitate this increase.

The benefits to people with nurses adopting the prescribing role are evident with improved clinical and health outcomes reported. Stakeholders are also satisfied with nurses adopting the prescribing role, with an increase in accessibility of services.

The developments in nurse prescribing necessitate quality prescribing educational resources and this book is such a resource. The book is superbly written and timely and I would like to congratulate Gould and Bain for such a compelling and comprehensive text.

It delivers essential prescribing knowledge for any nurse on the prescribing programme or for those qualified to prescribe. Educators will also find the book helpful for developing prescribing curricula. Various aspects of the prescribing process are addressed in each chapter with activities integrated throughout to help readers apply prescribing knowledge to practice. Chapters are fully referenced and the authors have provided a further reading list, including useful websites.

Professor Molly Courtenay
Professor of Health Sciences
Cardiff University

Introduction

About this book/who is this book for?

This textbook on the principles and practice of prescribing is written for pre-registration nursing students in all fields of practice, student midwives and health professionals who are undertaking prescribing programmes as part of their continuing development.

Why Principles and Practice of Nurse Prescribing?

The Nursing and Midwifery Council (NMC, 2018a) Code expects all registrants to:

> *prescribe, advise on, or provide medicines or treatment, including repeat prescriptions (only if you are suitably qualified) if you have enough knowledge of that person's health and are satisfied that the medicines or treatment serve that person's health needs.*

Prescribing by level one registered nurses has evolved considerably over the last 20 years. The **NMC** (2018b) standards for proficiency for the future nurse have an ambition for the newly qualified nurse to be prescribing ready at the point of registration. Within the first year of qualification, they could potentially undertake a prescribing qualification to prescribe from a limited formulary. Furthermore, after being qualified for one year, a registered nurse or midwife can progress to undertake a prescribing course that will allow them to prescribe from the full British National Formulary (**BNF**), with the exception of some specific controlled drugs (NMC, 2018c). Becoming a prescriber is by no means automatic and it is essential that the governance structures are in place to enable practitioners to undertake and be adequately supported throughout a prescribing programme (NMC, 2018c).

Prescribing related proficiencies have been identified to enable undergraduate nurses to be 'prescribing ready' at the point of registration. To progress to a prescribing qualification, the NMC (2018c) have adopted the Competency Framework for all prescribers (Royal Pharmaceutical Society (**RPS**)). This **RPS** framework was originally published by the National Prescribing Centre/National Institute for Health and Clinical Excellence in 2012, was updated by the RPS in 2016 for all regulators and professional bodies and was reviewed again in 2021. This book will therefore consider the NMC Future Nurse: Standards of Proficiency for Registered Nurses (NMC, 2018b), Standards for Prescribing Programmes (NMC, 2018d) and the RPS (2021a) Competency Framework for All Prescribers.

Book structure

This book is structured so that it will help you to understand and meet selected NMC proficiencies for the future nurse and address the RPS (2021a) Competency Framework for prescribers. The book has eight chapters and each chapter has a range of activities for you to reflect on your practice and support the application of theory to practice. The relevant proficiencies and competencies are presented at the start of each chapter so you can clearly see which ones are addressed.

Chapter 1 provides an overview of the professional context of prescribing. This chapter is framed around the Nursing and Midwifery Council (NMC) standards and the Royal Pharmaceutical Society's Competency Framework for All Prescribers, and provides an overview of the policy context and history. The de Silva family is introduced who will be used as a case study within many of the chapters.

Chapter 2 explores some of the underpinning legislation concerning prescribing. The importance of knowing your limitations and prescribing within your scope of practice is highlighted. Consent, mental capacity and autonomy are explored in relation to prescribing for adults and children and the requirements of a legal prescription are outlined. Ethical principles underpinning prescribing practice are explored.

Chapter 3 outlines a systematic approach to the process of decision-making as requiring a structured approach. A new model, RAPID-CASE, to aid prescribing decisions which integrates the features from consultation models, the original 'prescribing pyramid' (NPC, 1999b) and the Competency Framework for all prescribers is introduced.

Chapter 4 explores the evidence base that underpins prescribing and aspects of its clinical governance. Practitioners need to be able to demonstrate they have underpinned their prescribing decisions with recognised, reliable and appropriate evidence sources.

Chapter 5 includes core pharmacology principles and encourages readers to explore various methods and further resources to help embed the learning. Specific pharmacological topics to be covered include: routes of administration; pharmacokinetics; pharmacodynamics; drug effects; and pharmacology across the lifespan.

Chapter 6 explores the public health role of nurse prescribers and considers the responsibilities of prescribers in the context of population health. Specific public health issues such as antimicrobial stewardship are discussed. Teamworking in the context of prescribing practice is also considered.

Chapter 7 applies a structured approach to demonstrate the assessment of one example condition that can be prescribed for from the Nurse Prescribers' Formulary. Additional scenarios are used to prompt critical thinking around some of the other items you may be prescribing in the future within the context of your scope of practice.

Chapter 8 considers your accountability and methods by which to keep up to date as a prescriber linked to the NMC revalidation requirements.

It is important to recognise that some of the chapters are interlinked. In particular, Chapter 7 provides a worked example based on the application of RAPID-CASE introduced in Chapter 3.

Learning features

Learning from reading text is not always easy. Therefore, to provide variety and to assist with the development of independent learning skills and the application of theory to practice, this book contains activities, case studies, scenarios, further reading, useful websites and other materials to enable you to participate in your own learning. You will need to develop your own study skills and 'learn how to learn' to get the best from the material. The book cannot provide all the answers – but instead provides a framework for your learning.

The activities in the book will in particular help you to make sense of, and learn about, the material being presented. Some activities ask you to reflect on aspects of practice, or your experience of it, or the people or situations you encounter. *Reflection* is an essential skill in nursing, and it helps you to understand the world around you and often to identify how things might be improved. Other activities will help you develop key graduate skills such as your ability to *think critically* about a topic in order to challenge received wisdom, or your ability to *research a topic and find appropriate information and evidence,* and to be able to *make decisions* using that evidence in situations that are often difficult and time-pressured.

All the activities require you to take a break from reading the text, think through the issues presented and carry out some independent study, possibly using the internet. Where appropriate, there are sample answers presented at the end of each chapter, and these will help you to understand more fully your own reflections and independent study. Academic study always requires independent work; attending lectures will never be enough to be successful on your programme, and these activities will help to deepen your knowledge and understanding of the issues under scrutiny and give you practice at working on your own.

You might want to think about completing these activities as part of your personal development plan (PDP) or portfolio. After completing the activity write it up in your PDP or portfolio in a section devoted to that particular skill, then look back over time to see how far you are developing. You may also wish to start a 'personal formulary' of medicines and products you have gained familiarity with and are comfortable with administering, providing advice about or prescribing (when you have the qualification). You can also do more of the activities for a key skill that you have identified a weakness in, which will help build your skill and confidence in this area.

This book also contains a glossary on page 173 to assist you with unfamiliar terms. Glossary terms are in bold in the first instance that they appear.

We hope you enjoy this book and that through engaging with the range of activities provided this prepares your transition to becoming a future prescriber.

Chapter 1

The policy and professional context of nurse prescribing

RPS Competency Framework for All Prescribers (2021a)

This chapter will address the following professional competencies:

- **Competency 8: Prescribe professionally**

NMC Future Nurse: Standards of Proficiency for Registered Nurses

This chapter will address the following platforms and proficiencies:

Platform 1: Being an accountable professional
At the point of registration, the registered nurse will be able to:

1.1   understand and act in accordance with The Code: Professional standards of practice and behaviour for nurses, midwives and nursing associates and fulfil all registration requirements.

Chapter aims

After reading this chapter, you will be able to:

- explain the pertinence and benefits of prescribing to professional nursing;
- outline the core professional standards underpinning prescribing;
- discuss the pertinence of the prescribing competence framework. (RPS, 2021a)

Introduction

Within the Nursing and Midwifery Council, The Code: Professional Standards of Practice and Behaviour for Nurses, Midwives and Nursing Associates (NMC, 2018a) it is recognised that nurses are required to:

> *Advise on, prescribe, supply, dispense or administer medicines within the limits of your training and competence, the law, our guidance and other relevant policies, guidance and regulations.*

However, prescribing is not within the scope of practice of everyone on the register. Nursing associates or level two registered nurses don't prescribe, but they may supply, dispense and administer medicines. Only nurses and midwives who have successfully completed a further qualification in prescribing following their registration can prescribe. Nurse and midwife proficiencies (NMC, 2018a, 2019a) aim to provide registrants with the knowledge and skills from which to continuously develop, for example by being equipped to progress to the prescribing qualification.

Prescribing by nurses was legally established in 1992 in the UK after reports suggested prescribing would improve efficiency and quality (DHSS, 1986; DoH, 1989). The legislation underpinning this development (detailed in Chapter 2) took six years to come into effect and, more than 25 years later, prescribing is well established with approximately 90,000 prescribers on the Nursing and Midwifery Council (NMC) register (Table 1.1, NMC, 2021).

With countries

Area	2017	2018	2019	2020	2021	5 year +/−
V100 / V150 Community Practitioner Nurse Prescriber						
United Kingdom	**40,612**	**40,748**	**40,879**	**41,049**	**41,301**	**+689**
England only	32,849	32,709	32,839	32,949	33,169	+320
Scotland only	3,421	3,506	3,397	3,370	3,323	−98
Wales only	2,620	2,763	2,836	2,912	2,969	+349
NI only	1,437	1,499	1,534	1,560	1,582	+145
V200 Extended Formulary Prescriber						
United Kingdom	**1,449**	**1,375**	**1,292**	**1,211**	**1,152**	**−297**
England only	1,243	1,187	1,113	1,045	990	−253
Scotland only	183	170	158	148	143	−40
Wales only	12	10	11	9	9	−3
NI only	2	2	2	2	2	0

Area	2017	2018	2019	2020	2021	5 year +/−
V300 Nurse Independent/Supplementary Prescriber						
United Kingdom	**36,983**	**40,041**	**43,717**	**47,899**	**50,693**	**+13,710**
England only	30,853	33,305	36,308	39,755	41,878	+11,025
Scotland only	3,914	4,336	4,762	5,221	5,641	+1,727
Wales only	1,318	1,477	1,612	1,762	1,903	+585
NI only	672	709	809	911	1,013	+341
TOTAL	**79,044**	**82,164**	**85,888**	**90,159**	**93,146**	**+14,102**
Please note: Some of the figures are lower than stated because registrants with different types of prescribing qualifications are counted twice						

Table 1.1   Number of prescribers in the NMC register (NMC, 2021)

As per Table 1.1, these prescribers are split between community practitioner nurse prescribers, known as V100 or V150 prescribers, who can prescribe from a limited formulary, and nurse independent prescribers, V300, who can prescribe from the full British National Formulary (BNF), with the exception of some specific controlled drugs (NMC, 2018c). The table also shows a decline in the V200 prescriber, a qualification which has been superseded by the V300 and is no longer available. This represents a steady expansion of professional autonomy and accountability with nurses and midwives now expected to have the skills to progress to a prescribing qualification immediately following registration (NMC, 2018c) and potentially undertake full formulary (V300) prescribing after one year post-registration experience. Some people are describing this as 'prescribing ready' at the point of registration.

Like most professional regulators, the Nursing and Midwifery Council sets standards of practice and education which enables entry onto the professional register as a nurse or midwife. Legal statutes give the NMC the authority to define both the requirements of educational programmes and the competencies or proficiencies that need to be achieved. The over-arching objective of the Council is the protection of the public, which is done by setting standards of education, training, conduct and performance and ensuring the maintenance of those standards.

Pre-registration nurses are measured against a number of outcomes within seven platforms (NMC, 2018b). Platform four relating to providing and evaluating care is explicit in that nurses must be able to *apply knowledge of pharmacology to the care of people, demonstrating the ability to progress to a prescribing qualification following registration* (NMC, 2018b, p12). Similarly, midwife proficiencies (NMC, 2019a, p21), divided into domains rather than platforms, state that at the point of registration midwives must demonstrate *knowledge and understanding of the principles of safe and effective administration and optimisation of prescription and non-prescription medicines and midwives exemptions, demonstrating the ability to progress to a prescribing qualification following registration.*

Annotation on the NMC register as a nurse or midwife prescriber requires the successful completion of an NMC approved post-registration prescribing programme in order to meet the necessary standards of prescribing programmes. Within these standards the NMC (2018c) has adopted the Royal Pharmaceutical Society (RPS) Competency Framework for All Prescribers as their proficiency standards for nurse prescribing. The revised version of the RPS Competency Framework was produced and adopted in 2021. The adoption of this Competency Framework demonstrates a commitment to an interdisciplinary approach to developing prescribing proficiency (NMC, 2018c). This book will therefore consider the NMC Future Nurse: Standards of Proficiency for Registered Nurses (NMC, 2018b), Standards for Prescribing Programmes (NMC, 2018e) and the RPS (2021a) Competency Framework for All Prescribers.

This chapter starts with a brief overview of the policy context, benefits and outline of the different types of prescribing qualifications. It then moves onto the topic of the standards and competencies relevant to nurse prescribing. While this embeds principles of safe and effective medicines management, the focus is on prescribing and, in particular, community practitioner nurse prescribing (coded on the NMC register as V100 and V150). Next, the RPS Competency Framework for All Prescribers will be discussed. This framework includes prescribing in relation to assessment and consultation, ethical issues, legal issues, professional issues, accountability, evidence-based practice, public health, team working, record keeping, pharmacology, prescription writing and numeracy. The chapter will end with a discussion of scope of practice.

Scenario 1.1

You work in a busy community nursing team and have recently moved to a health centre so are no longer GP attached. You have visited Mrs A and assessed her as needing some new dressings, paracetamol and BM (blood sugar) testing strips. In the past, you would have printed off the prescription and asked the GP to sign it so it could be processed that day. However, now that your team has moved, the GPs are refusing to do this. You ask the district nurse to write the prescription as she has the prescribing qualification. However, she says she is not able to prescribe unless she has assessed the patient.

A brief history of nurse prescribing

The need for nurses to prescribe first became apparent in a review of community nursing services in the 1980s. Similar to Scenario 1.1, as part of the review of 'neighbourhood nursing' (DHSS, 1986) Baroness Cumberlege witnessed 'well-informed and qualified nurses' standing outside GPs' doors to get prescriptions signed, sometimes having written the prescription themselves (Cumberlege, 2003, p10). The review team was also alarmed to find that house-bound people were waiting in pain and discomfort for the prescription they needed, with particularly lengthy delays in some areas. Nurse prescribing was a logical response to an identified health need and to some extent the authorisation of existing practice.

Throughout the gradual development of nurse prescribing, there have been mixed views from other professional organisations. The initial recommendations were modest as they 'anticipated the hostility from both the medical and pharmaceutical professions' (Cumberlege, 2003, p12). Initially, prescribing was approved for only specialist community practitioners (health visitors and district nurses) from a limited choice of items contained in a Nurse Prescribers' Formulary (NPF). This is now known as V100 prescribing, when the programme is undertaken within a district nurse or specialist community public health programme; or V150 if undertaken as a standalone programme by any qualified nurse or midwife. After legislation was passed, nurse prescribing was piloted in England in 1994, followed by its introduction in the other UK countries. The legislation in Scotland to allow district nurses, health visitors and practice nurses with a recognised qualification to prescribe from a limited formulary was passed in 1996 (The National Health Service (pharmaceutical services) (Scotland), (General Medical supplies) (Scotland), and (Charges for Drugs and Appliances) (Scotland) Amendment Regulations). Subsequent expansion of prescribing rights has been achieved in incremental stages assisted by a variety of mechanisms across the four UK countries including research, audit, service evaluation and consultation (Latter *et al.*, 2005a, 2005b; MHRA, 2005, 2006; i5 Health, 2015).

Activity 1.1 will prompt you to think critically about the introduction of nurse prescribing and what it has meant for the profession.

Activity 1.1   Critical thinking: benefits of nurse prescribing

Thinking about your practice, what are some of the benefits of prescribing from a limited formulary or having a wider scope to prescribe? What do you think the research, audits and evaluation have shown? What do you think may be some of the disadvantages or challenges of its introduction?

A selection of findings from qualitative studies and reviews of nurse prescribing can be found at the end of this chapter.

As you will have seen in the answer to Activity 1.1, since its inception nurse prescribing has consistently evaluated as safe and effective, with improved patient outcomes reported (Latter and Courtenay, 2004; Latter *et al.*, 2005a; Holmes, 2006; DoH, 2006a, b; Latter *et al.*, 2010). This success combined with health policies expanding nursing roles resulted in the series of extensions to the initial programme. In May 2001, following the recommendations of the 2nd Crown Report (DoH, 1999) and a consultation period, the government announced that nurse prescribing would be extended to more nurses and a wider range of medicines, to include: minor ailments; minor injuries; health promotion; and palliative care. An accompanying educational programme was developed and approved by the Nursing and Midwifery Council (NMC). This was known as 'Extended Formulary Prescribing' and denoted by the NMC as V200.

In 2003 legislation changed to allow nurses and pharmacists to also become supplementary prescribers. Nurses that had previously completed the V200 were provided an opportunity to 'top up' their qualification to become independent and supplementary prescribers. It was at this point from an NMC perspective that the prescribing qualification was known as V300 prescribing. After another national consultation process, further changes to regulations allowed nurses and pharmacists to be able to prescribe any licensed medicine for any medical condition they are competent to treat, including a limited range of controlled drugs for specific medical conditions (DoH, 2006a). Additional amendments to legislation in relation to the professional use of controlled drugs by pharmacists and nurses came into force in 2012 and apply in Scotland, England and Wales. The increased importance of nurse prescribing is evident in health policy (DoH, 2006c, 2009; NHS England, 2019; Scottish Government, 2017), with the remit of providing services closer to the patient, the extension of nursing (and other professionals') roles and the emphasis on a proactive approach to health and wellbeing (Scottish Government, 2016; DHSC, 2021a, b).

Nurse prescribing continues to develop at a considerable rate and it is therefore important that you regularly access relevant websites to keep abreast of new developments. It is worth remembering that the power and responsibility to develop and implement policy within health services were devolved to the Scottish Executive and Welsh Assembly. Therefore, what is contained within the Department of Health's website does not always apply throughout the UK. It is important that you take cognisance of these factors when undertaking your reading as publications prior to 2006 will not reflect the current situation, although will still contain valuable theories and principles. The timeline in Figure 1.1 illustrates the development of nurse and midwife prescribing, some of which will be explored further later in the book. Although NMC Standards and Competency Frameworks are the same across the four countries, each has different policies affecting prescribing. The initial Acts for nurse and midwife prescribing indicate these separate dates for all four countries, while dates of further development are mainly based on English law.

Types of prescribers

The Nursing and Midwifery Council (2018e) prescribing standards have consolidated a number of circulars and previous standards. The following types of prescribers and their associated codes are outlined in Table 1.2.

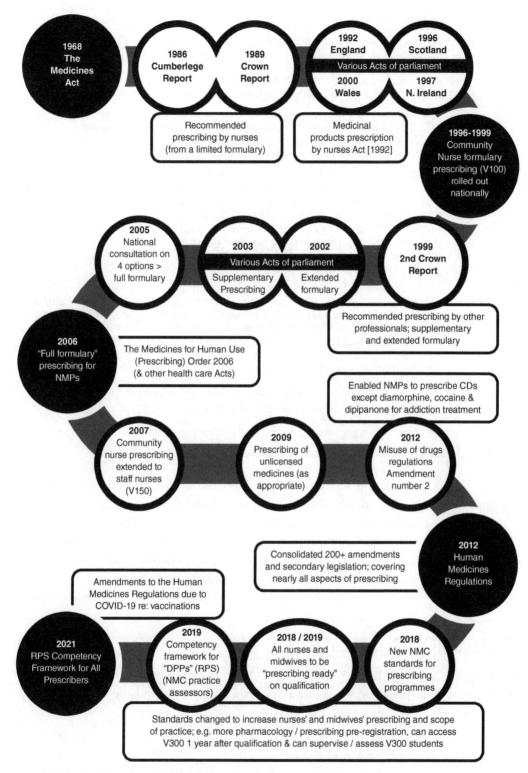

Figure 1.1 Prescribing timeline

NMC Code	Title Description	Formulary
V100	Community practitioner nurse prescriber. As part of the Specialist Qualification Practice (SPQ) (District Nursing/General Practice Nursing, etc.) standards or taught within a Specialist Community Public Health Nursing course (health visitors, school nurses, etc.)	Nurse Prescriber's Formulary
V150	Community practitioner nurse or midwife prescriber; prescribing from the Nurse Prescriber's Formulary; as a standalone course, not linked to a specialist, public health or other post-registration nursing programme	Nurse Prescriber's Formulary
V200	Nurse or midwife independent prescriber who initially was only able to prescribe from an extended formulary, prior to the changes in legislation in 2003 to include supplementary prescribing. V200 prescribers can now prescribe as independent prescribers on the same basis as V300 prescribers but are not able to act as supplementary prescribers. The V200 prescribing programmes are no longer offered	British National Formulary (with the exception of some controlled drugs)
V300	Nurse or midwife independent and supplementary prescriber; the current qualification for all prescribing courses for nurses or midwives who can prescribe any medicine for any condition within their competence with the exception of some controlled drugs (for the purposes of addiction treatment). V300 also includes supplementary prescribing which is for those who choose to work in partnership with a doctor or dentist to implement a clinical management plan in agreement with the individual being prescribed for; and allows all drugs to be prescribed within the CMP	British National Formulary (with the exception of some controlled drugs) as independent prescriber; and full British National Formulary as supplementary prescriber

Table 1.2   Types of nurse and midwife prescribers

The two main types of prescribing (V100/V150 and V300) entail different programmes of study to be approved by the Nursing and Midwifery Council. While the NMC (2018c) standards for education are less detailed than previous, they outline different entry criteria between the two courses and specify that a pharmacology and a calculations exam are required. Both courses involve achieving the same competencies contained in the Competency Framework for All Prescribers (RPS, 2021a).

Professional Standards

The NMC Code (NMC 2018a) statement 18.1 sets out common standards of conduct and behaviour for nurses on the register and expects all registrants to:

prescribe, advise on, or provide medicines or treatment, including repeat prescriptions (only if you are suitably qualified) if you have enough knowledge of that person's health and are satisfied that the medicines or treatment serve that person's health needs.

Prior to entering the register individuals will undertake an NMC approved education programme to achieve the required outcomes. There are 103 pre-registration nursing standard statements on seven 'platforms' and 188 midwifery standard statements across six domains. As outlined previously, the expectation upon registration for both is to be able to demonstrate the ability to progress to a prescribing qualification following registration (NMC, 2018b, 2019a). If registrants choose to progress to a prescribing qualification and undertake a further preparation programme the NMC (2018e) states:

> *For all categories of prescribers, the RPS Competency Framework applies in full and demonstration of all those competencies contained within it must be achieved in order to be awarded prescriber status.* (NMC, 2018e, p5)

A Competency Framework for All Prescribers (CFAP) (RPS, 2021a)

A previous Competency Framework for prescribers was published in 2012, by the National Prescribing Centre/National Institute for Health and Clinical Excellence (NICE) to support all prescribers to prescribe effectively. It was recognised that a common framework was needed, whether the prescriber was a medical doctor, nurse, pharmacist or other allied health professional, due to the challenges associated with safe and effective prescribing. **NICE** have backed the RPS in updating the framework in collaboration with all the prescribing professions UK wide. The updated Competency Framework for All Prescribers (CFAP) was first published for all regulators, professional bodies, prescribing professions in 2016 and an overview of the development process is available on the Royal Pharmaceutical Society's website. As it is important for competency frameworks to reflect current practice, it is reviewed at regular intervals, with a revised version consulted upon and published in 2021. NMC approved prescribing programmes will be expected to embed the most current version of the CFAP.

The NMC (2018b) reminds that these competencies also need to be maintained after the qualification is achieved and the CFAP (RPS, 2021a) is used for the initial prescribing programme as well as to structure ongoing development as a prescriber. There are 76 prescribing competency statements across ten core areas (RPS, 2021a). Many of these competencies overlap with outcomes nurses are expected to achieve at the point of registration, although at that point nurses cannot legally prescribe (NMC, 2018e). Undertaking a thorough assessment to underpin safe decision-making for the individuals in your care is one of the key considerations whether a prescribing decision is made or not (NMC, 2018a, 2018e; RPS, 2021a).

The steps to prescribing competence

The visual accompanying the RPS (2021a) competencies shows the person (being prescribed for) in the centre surrounded by two layers of prescribing. For a more practical interpretation, the broad competencies (RPS, 2021a) are depicted in Figure 1.2 as a stepped approach to prescribing. This model starts with clinical governance-related competences at the base recognising that governance forms the foundation of professional considerations from which you can proceed on the prescribing journey. An episode of prescribing will finish with governance as well, for example, in documentation, reflecting on your prescribing decisions and undertaking continuing professional development.

As a nurse, governance is underpinned by the Code (NMC, 2018a). For example, the principles of only prescribing within your scope of practice and competence, accepting responsibility and understanding the legal and ethical implications of prescribing are considered first. While some of the prescribing governance competencies are concerned with improving prescribing practice, they broadly cover topics that are before or after encounters with people for whom you may be prescribing. Like the RPS (2021a) visual, these 'steps to prescribing competence' in Figure 1.2 also place the person at the centre of your practice, as a reminder that they should be considered *at every step* of the process. While this model includes all ten broad competency statements, a more practical consultation model (RAPID-CASE) is introduced in Chapter 3 as a way to logically frame your assessment and decision-making for individuals in your care.

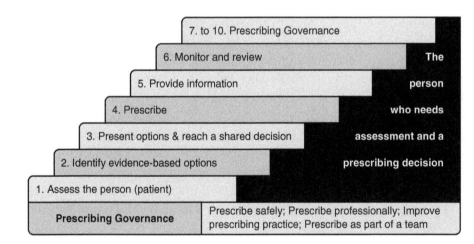

Figure 1.2   The steps to prescribing competence (based on RPS, 2021a)

Activity 1.2   Reflection

Thinking about your practice, what are some of the models, tools, frameworks you currently use to inform your practice? What would be the benefits from using a model designed for prescribing competence? What would be the barriers?

There is no answer provided for Activity 1.2, but this will be further explored as you progress through Chapter 3.

Applying the framework

We have outlined some of the professional requirements of prescribing courses and the framework containing the competencies that need to be achieved. Applying the steps to prescribing competence is illustrated in the chapters to follow by using a fictitious family (Activity 1.3: Scenario). The characters within this scenario are revisited throughout the book with the aim of exploring a variety of decision-making or prescribing situations across the life span.

Activity 1.3   Scenario: the de Silva family

Mohammad (Mo) and Cathryn (Cath) have been married for ten years and have three children living at home. Cath's dad passed away recently and he was the main carer for her mum (Mrs Fiona Smith), an 84-year-old who has mild dementia and now lives with the family. Mo is currently unemployed, with minor health problems, although he has smoked for 20 years and is prone to coughs and colds. Cath is normally well, but has found life more challenging since their third child, especially with her mum living with them. Sana is their 15-year-old daughter and is still in school, Sam is four years old and has just started infant school, while Milly has just turned six weeks.

The needs of this family will be explored in the context of an example professional role (e.g. as a health visitor, school nurse, practice nurse, staff nurse or district nurse).

In this instance, you are a health visitor who is undertaking the six-week review. While you are there, Cath asks you to prescribe some paracetamol for her mum. She says she doesn't have time to take her to the doctors' surgery and she thinks her leg wound is playing up.

Starting with the bottom step, what are some of the governance aspects of this request that you would need to consider?

Possible answers to this activity can be found at the end of this chapter and further elements of this model will be explored in subsequent chapters.

Chapter summary

This chapter explored the historic development of prescribing leading up to current standards of education and competence. An overview of the timeline and types of prescribing were discussed. The prescribing competence framework was presented alongside an adapted model to aid future prescribing decisions. To put this model in context the de Silva family were introduced as an example scenario that can be revisited bearing in mind

(Continued)

(Continued)

the steps to prescribing competence. In this instance, prescribing governance needs to be at the forefront and act as the basis for which prescribing practice can be developed. The next chapter explores these principles to a greater depth in relation to the legal and ethical aspects of prescribing.

Activities: suggested answers and discussion points

Answer to Activity 1.1 Critical thinking: benefits of nurse prescribing

The benefits of nurse prescribing have been demonstrated through ongoing research and reviews.

Benefits

- *Safe and effective:* There is considerable evidence that NMP not only has a very strong safety record but provides significant advantages to patients and the NHS as a whole (i5 Health, 2015).
- *Nurse prescribing has consistently been evaluated as safe and effective with improved patient outcomes:* Luker *et al.* (1997, 1998), DoH (2005), Latter and Courtenay (2004), Latter *et al.* (2005a, 2005b, 2010, 2011), Holmes (2006).
- *Improved patient outcomes:* Luker *et al.* (1998), Mundinger *et al.* (2000), Franklin (2006), i5 Health (2015).
- *Autonomy:* Less dependence on doctors/increased autonomy for practitioners: Luker *et al.*, 1997).
- *Improved concordance:* DoH, 2002a, 2004.
- *Cost-effective:* i5 Health, 2015.

Disadvantages/areas for concern

- *Increased responsibility/accountability:* Luker *et al.* (1997).
- *Pharmacological knowledge of nurses:* Latter *et al.* (2004).
- *Ongoing support/CPD:* i5 Health (2015, p20) found there was a significant minority of pre-scribers who mentioned a need for more support or that had experienced difficulty in accessing training and support.
- *Constraints:* Prescribers reported several issues impacting on their ability to prescribe effectively (i5 Health, 2015).

Answer to Activity 1.3 Scenario: the de Silva family

The NMC (2018a, e) are clear that you are not permitted to prescribe until you have completed a recognised course and the qualification has been annotated on the professional record. In this scenario, even with the qualification, as part of the competence to prescribe safely you need to be sure to only prescribe within your own scope of practice and recognise the limits of own knowledge and skill. Although it can be argued this is an over the counter medication, as opposed to a prescription-only medication, a skilled assessment should be always be undertaken (explored more fully in Chapter 3).

Other professional principles include the need to accept personal responsibility for prescribing and understanding the legal and ethical implications. In this instance, it may also be unclear who Mrs Smith is registered with so access to records could be an issue. While this request may not be currently in your remit, the professional principle of acting as part of a multidisciplinary team, communicating effectively and aiming to ensure continuity of care across care settings is also pertinent. This may involve establishing relationships with other professionals based on understanding, trust and respect for each other's roles in relation to prescribing, whether with the district nurse, or general practitioner or other involved in her care.

Further reading and useful websites

This chapter introduced some of the professional considerations of prescribing. These core resources are recommended to support your journey as a professional developing your prescribing.

The core source of medicines information is the British National Formulary. This is published every six months in hard copy, with the online version or app updated more frequently. The hard copy version may go out of date more quickly, but it has additional content compared with the online sources, so is highly recommended as a comprehensive information source. For prescribing purposes, you must always use the most up-to-date version, or check for changes via alerts, or the online/app versions. There is a separate BNF for Children (BNFc) and a Nurse Prescribers Formulary (NPF).

- Joint Formulary Committee (JFC) *British National Formulary* (online). London: BMJ Group and Pharmaceutical Press. https://bnf.nice.org.uk
- The British National Formulary for Children (BNFc). https://bnfc.nice.org.uk
- Community Practitioner Nurse Prescribers Formulary (NPF). https://bnf.nice.org.uk/nurse-prescribers-formulary/

The Nursing and Midwifery Council has a variety of pertinent information including the professional standards, information about CPD and a series of guides for practice assessors and supervisors. It is recommended to start with the standards.

- Main website. https://www.nmc.org.uk/
- Post-registration Standards (for Prescribers). https://www.nmc.org.uk/standards/standards-for-post-registration/

The NMC standards for medicines management were withdrawn in 2019, so the RCN information on this topic is recommended. It can be found on the RCN website for prescribers, along with selected resources.

- RCN: Medicines Management. https://www.rcn.org.uk/clinical-topics/medicines-management
- RCN: Advice Guide Non-medical prescribers. https://www.rcn.org.uk/get-help/rcn-advice/non-medical-prescribers

The Royal Pharmaceutical Society (RPS) publishes competency frameworks for prescribers, and their supervisors/assessors (DPPs). These frameworks, along with further resources for a range of professionals, are available from the RPS website.

- RPS Competency Framework. https://www.rpharms.com/resources/frameworks/prescribers-competency-framework
- RPS Medicines Optimisation Hub. https://www.rpharms.com/resources/pharmacy-guides/medicines-optimisation-hub

Chapter 2 — The legal and ethical context of nurse prescribing

Chapter aims

After reading this chapter, you will be able to:

- explain legal accountability and duty of care as a prescriber;

- outline core legislation underpinning prescribing and prescription writing;
- explore ethical concepts of pertinence to your prescribing practice.

Introduction

Scenario

You are a new graduate who has just joined a small nursing team. First impressions are they seem stressed and the team leader has criticised your documentation several times. You discover the nurse you replaced has gone off work with stress due to an ongoing coroner's case where a prescribing incident resulted in harm.

As a professional and as a prescriber you hold accountability for your actions or omissions. When things go wrong, harm may come to the people in your care and this can affect you as well as those around you. The transition to a qualified prescriber brings greater accountability legally, ethically and professionally. Prescribing practice was explored in the professional context in Chapter 1 and is now looked at more closely, with a focus on legal and ethical implications.

Professionalism, law and ethics are closely linked, with some of the core concepts overlapping. For example, 'duty of care' embedded in professional standards (NMC, 2018a) is also a recognised legal concept (Griffith, 2019) and underpins ethical principles (Beauchamp and Childress, 2019). An overview of some of these are provided, while their significance and application should be explored further within your area and scope of practice. As it is never a valid legal defence to claim that you were unaware of a particular law, attention to the legal implications of prescribing is a professional expectation also needed to safely expand your practice. Ways to help address legal requirements include employment law (indemnity, vicarious liability), engaging with mandatory training, adhering to professional standards, working within your area of recognised competence and keeping your knowledge and skills up to date.

This chapter starts with an outline of the various sources of accountability before focusing on selected laws of pertinence to prescribing and the legal authority to prescribe. This includes reference to some acts of law that apply more broadly to professional practice, such as duty of care and consent and capacity. The link between consent, mental capacity and autonomy is explored in relation to prescribing for adults and children and the requirements of a legal prescription are outlined. The chapter closes with a discussion of ethical principles underpinning prescribing practice, with a focus on the implications for your decision-making.

Accountability and error

People requiring healthcare are known to experience harm, particularly by the medications that are intended as their treatment. Unsafe medication practices and medication errors are a leading cause of injury and avoidable harm in healthcare systems across the world (WHO, 2017). Elliot *et al.* (2018) echo this and highlight that medication error can cause increased use of healthcare services and varying degrees of harm, including death. There isn't a consensus on the specific number, but Barnett *et al.* (2011) suggest that between 5 and 20 per cent of all hospital admissions are due to medications.

- A detailed 'rapid review' into medication errors by Elliot *et al.* (2018, p16) estimated that in excess of 237,396,371 medication errors occur in England per annum, at all stages of medication use and in all settings.
- Of these, *72.1% are classed as minor with little or no potential for clinical harm,* while the other 61.4 million and 4.8 million errors respectively have potential to cause moderate or severe harm.
- Of these 66.2 million clinically significant errors, 47 million occur in primary care, of which 22.5 million in prescribing.
- In respect to the economic burden Elliot *et al.* (2018, p4) estimate the NHS costs of *definitely avoidable ADRs are £98.5 million per year, consuming 181,626 bed-days, causing 712 deaths, and contributing to 1,708 deaths.*

Whether as a prescriber or more broadly as a healthcare practitioner there is a clear case for being aware of your accountability in relation to medications and the steps you can take to protect the people in your care, your colleagues and yourself. Practitioners can be seen as a 'second victim' because of the impact of making errors. Klein *et al.* (2017, p771) assert that medical students should develop strategies for coping with error as it has been found that doctors can experience *guilt, shame, fear, humiliation, loss of confidence, deep concerns about their professional skills and social isolation.* As your autonomy increases, so too does the risk of error and the need to be prepared.

Coping with the challenges of practice and the possibility of inadvertently causing harm, is helped by always being aware of your accountability, taking ownership for the effects of your acts or omissions, working within your scope of practice and recognising your own limitations and development needs. As professionals, we are held accountable in a number of ways, as illustrated in Figure 2.1. Activity 2.1 asks you to think critically about your accountability in these four areas.

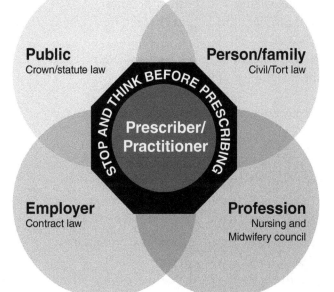

Figure 2.1 Four areas of accountability

Activity 2.1 Critical thinking

You are a recently qualified nurse who has started a new job in a busy GP practice. You have been asked to run a wound care clinic and make treatment decisions for wounds with a variety of causes and underlying conditions. Some of the clinical presentations are new to you and you find there isn't always someone available to ask for assistance. Thinking about the four main areas of accountability in Figure 2.1, outline how you would be held to account if harm occurred to one of the people in your care. What strategies could you take to minimise the risk of this happening?

An outline answer is to be found at the end of the chapter.

Four areas of accountability

As you have found in Activity 2.1, the four spheres of accountability can overlap and have their own requirements that need to be met. An extreme example from practice could be seen as the deliberately harmful administration of medicines by a nurse who was found guilty of murdering two patients and causing grievous bodily harm to several more. Due to his actions and their impact, this nurse was held to account by all four areas of the law.

- **Civil**: (litigation/negligence/tort law) his employing health authority paid compensation to the victims and/or their families.
- **Criminal**: (Crown prosecution) he was charged in a criminal court for murder and grievous bodily harm.
- **Professional**: he was struck off the professional NMC register.
- **Employment**: he was dismissed from his job.

Each of these are explored in further detail:

- **Civil**: (litigation/negligence/tort law) Tort law is most commonly associated with compensation for harm that has occurred through acts or omissions. It is linked to 'negligence' with Griffith (2019) suggesting it is best defined as 'actionable harm'. Griffith (2019) explains that court rulings over the years have established that successful negligence cases require these three key features:
  1. the patient was owed a duty of care by the practitioner;
  2. there was a breach of that duty of care; and
  3. the breach of duty caused loss or harm recognised by the courts.

- **Criminal**: (Crown prosecution) For an action or omission to be considered a crime, the same requirements of the civil case must be met, but it also needs to be seen as a crime by the state and normally have an element of premeditation or intent involved. The legal test is more stringent, with intent to harm needing to be proven, although the laws were augmented in 2015 [Criminal Justice and Courts Act, 2015], so more cases can be tried in a criminal court than previously. An early example of this was the case of two nurses found guilty of wilful neglect when they admitted falsifying BM (blood glucose) results that were being used to calculate insulin dosages (Bolton, 2015). They were sentenced to eight months in prison, lost their jobs and were struck off the NMC register (Griffith, 2018).

- **Professional**: Professional accountability means that practitioners subject to successful prosecution for civil or criminal misconduct are likely to be removed from their professional register. As professional regulators, such as the NMC, aim to protect patients and promote public trust in their nursing professionals, removal from the register can also result from hearings for serious breaches of professional conduct. Professional regulators have a statutory duty to the public, with acts of law defining the boundaries of their authority and remit. For example, the NMC has the power to admit or remove practitioners from the register, annotate additional qualifications and define educational and practice standards [Article 19(6) of the Nursing and Midwifery Order 2001].

- **Employment**: Accountability is addressed by the signing of an employment contract, and practitioners are protected by employers' vicarious liability. In this way, the employer takes indirect responsibility for the actions of practitioners carrying out their contracted duties. Extra responsibilities, such as prescribing, should be added to job descriptions if it is a role requirement and professional indemnity is required. The addition of these extra duties to employment contracts helps to make responsibilities and duties clear and consequently support vicarious liability.

Duty of care

All professionals owe a 'duty of care' to the people in their care. It refers to the legal obligation to always act in a person's best interest, to ensure no act or omission results in harm and to act safely within your competence. From that starting point, the consequences of breaching duty of care such as negligence, ill-treatment or wilful neglect can occur.

> In the case of R(Burke) v GMC [2005], Lord Diplock outlined a duty of care as a: *single comprehensive duty covering all the ways you are called on to exercise skill and judgement in improving the mental and physical condition of the patient.*

When you owe a duty of care to a person in your care there is a legal requirement to ensure your decisions (whether actions or omissions) do not cause them harm (Griffith and Tengnah, 2017). Clinical negligence is when people are physically or mentally harmed because of the standard of healthcare provided. While each case is judged individually, examples of potential negligence include:

- a failure to assess symptoms adequately, making an incorrect diagnosis, ruling out or missing a diagnosis;
- discharging someone too early, offering poor advice or inadequate follow-up care;
- prescribing the wrong medication or treatment.

For many years, the legal case determining if the action or omission was below the expected standard was the Bolam v Friern Hospital Management Committee [1957], often referred to as the 'Bolam test'. The principle is that a professional is *not guilty of negligence if he has acted in accordance with a practice accepted as proper by a responsible body of medical men skilled in that particular art* (Bolam v Friern HMC 1957). The Bolam test is now thought to be at risk of subjectivity. The later Bolitho v City & Hackney Health Authority [1997] ruling indicated the body of expert opinion should be able to demonstrate the standard of care has a logical basis, particularly in the weighing of risks against benefits.

The implication for prescribers is being able to articulate a defensible rationale for their clinical judgements. This reflects an increased emphasis on guidelines, research and evidence-based decision-making in the health service. Griffith (2019, p37) suggests that although *the law is generally content to allow the profession to set its standards of care, it reserves the right to reject a standard that does not stand up to logical analysis.* This was seen to be a clear change from the standard of care being what was 'accepted practice' to that standard being based on 'expected practice' (Samanta and Samanta, 2003). Relatedly, another milestone case (Montgomery vs Lanarkshire Health Board, 2015) addresses the duty of care with regard to the disclosure of information to people, in particular in relation to the risks of recommended treatments and other options.

> The landmark UK Supreme Court judgement in Montgomery v Lanarkshire Health Board [2015, p28] ruled that the standard of care requires practitioners to take *reasonable care to ensure that the patient is aware of any material risks involved in any recommended treatment, and of any reasonable alternative or variant treatments.*

A sound knowledge of the risks, benefits and evidence base underpinning clinical practice is integral to providing informed treatment options and advice. This aligns with a person-centred approach to prescribing practice. Health policy generally promotes person-centred care, and the RPS (2021a) competencies specifically refer to shared decision-making and 'providing information' reflecting this legal ruling. Your duty of care as a prescriber requires you to act carefully in your assessment and treatment decisions, be able to logically justify these actions and show that the people in your care have been informed of the risks and benefits of the recommended treatments. While the ambition is for informed choice, time pressures, communication barriers and other practical challenges may influence your decision-making. Some of these are addressed in Activity 2.2 and through the discussion of consent, autonomy and mental capacity in the sections to follow. Activity 2.2 asks you to critically consider your duty of care in relation to informed choice for treatment decisions.

Activity 2.2   Critical thinking: duty of care – informed choice

There is an expectation that working within the RPS (2021a) competencies, practising professionally and within the law, you will promote informed choice. When prescribing medicines or other products, what might be some of the barriers to informed choice?

An outline of possible answers (presented as biomedical or psycho-social) can be found at the end of the chapter.

Duty of care: consent and autonomy

Activity 2.2 offered challenges to your duty of care to promote autonomy and informed decision-making. Practitioners have a professional and legal duty to obtain a person's consent to discharge their duty of care. Consent is in relation to any actions such as assessment, treatment, care or advice provided, as well as for using a person's information. The NMC (2018a) reminds that 'properly informed consent' must be obtained and documented before carrying out any action. Practitioners need to be aware of laws relating to mental capacity while ensuring that the rights and best interests are upheld for those who are assessed as lacking capacity (NMC, 2018a). The RPS (2021a) framework includes consent in one of the competencies along with confidentiality, dignity and safeguarding.

> The National Institute for Health and Care Excellence (NICE) (2018a, p31) define consent as the: *voluntary and continuing permission of the person to receive particular treatment or care and support, based on an adequate knowledge of the purpose, nature, likely effects and risks including the likelihood of success, any alternatives to it and what will happen if the treatment does not go ahead.*

Consent can also have a clinical purpose in increasing the likelihood of confidence in and cooperation with the treatment. Legally, without consent a practitioner can be charged with 'ill-treatment', 'assault' or 'trespass to the person' (Griffith and Tengnah, 2011). The principle underpinning consent is that of self-determination or the right to choose how to live one's life. Medicines and other treatments are implicated in this right to determine, meaning that people retain the legal right to accept or decline these. The implication for prescribers and those tasked with administering medications is that even with a prescription (or other authority to administer a medicine) the person must consent and has the legal right to refuse medicines (Griffith, 2015). For consent to be valid, Griffith and Tengnah (2011) explain, it needs to be *full, free* and *reasonably informed*.

1. **Full**: This involves gaining consent for all the treatments being proposed. An example of this is a surgical case where a patient had a potentially harmful lump removed while undergoing another procedure. However, as prior consent had not been obtained for removing the lump the surgeon was found guilty of trespass (Williamson v East London & City HA [1998]).
2. **Free**: (voluntary) As consent is an act of autonomy it must be the free choice of the individual and not obtained by undue influence. While nurses may have legitimate influence, in law this must not limit the person's free will or force their choices and we should also be alert to undue influence by family members (Griffith and Tengnah, 2011). Prescribers must be certain that the choice being made is that of the patient and not the external control of others.
3. **Informed**: Valid consent requires that health professionals explain what the treatment entails and explain the risks (Sidaway v Bethlem Royal Hospital [1985]). The ruling in Montgomery vs Lanarkshire [2015] expands on past cases and implies that not only must adequate information be given regarding what the treatment involves and its benefits and risks, but also whether there are sensible alternatives, and the implications of no treatment.

Expressed and implied consent

As a professional or prescriber, you need to ensure consent is obtained and this can be in one of two ways: expressed, or implied. Expressed can be verbal or written, while implied is the interpretation of the person's actions, which must be documented. While valid consent is needed for each episode of care and treatment (Griffith and Tengnah, 2011), prescribers are not 'obliged to provide treatment they do not believe to be clinically indicated, so a patient cannot demand healthcare' (Griffith and Tengnah, 2012, p.142).

Duty of care: consent and mental capacity

The requirements for valid consent are outlined above, with the implication that the person being treated understands the information being provided. They must be deemed capable of giving consent for the specified action(s), which requires the assessment of mental capacity. Having the mental capacity to consent means they understand the information given to them, can demonstrate this understanding and can use it to make an informed decision. Without capacity to consent, the principle of best interest applies. Where people are unable to give or express consent, the Mental Capacity Act (MCA) [2005] provides the legal framework for acting and making decisions on their behalf. The MCA Code of Practice (Department for Constitutional Affairs (DCA), 2007, p15) states the underlying philosophy of the MCA is *to ensure that any decision made, or action taken, on behalf of someone who lacks the capacity to make the decision or act for themselves is made in their best interests.*

When assessing a person's decision-making capacity a two-stage test should be used. This involves establishing:

- if the person has an impairment of the mind or brain, or is there some sort of disturbance affecting the way their mind or brain works (it doesn't matter whether this is temporary or permanent);
- if so, does that impairment or disturbance mean that the person is unable to make the decision in question at the time it needs to be made.

While these questions apply for all types of treatment decisions, some examples of pertinence for prescribing include assuring the person understands:

- the examination or diagnostic procedures required;
- the risks and benefits, **cautions** or interactions of treatment;
- the instructions for storage and administration;
- requirements for monitoring and how to seek advice/support.

The MCA Code (DCA, 2007, p45) outlines that a person is unable to make a decision if they cannot:

1. understand information about the decision to be made (the Act calls this 'relevant information');

2. retain that information in their mind;
3. use or weigh that information as part of the decision-making process; or
4. communicate their decision (by talking, sign language or any other means).

This is of pertinence to prescribing, as you will encounter people who may be able to make certain decisions (e.g. consent to your assessment), but not others, such as retain the information needed to safely take the prescribed treatment. As the aim is to promote the best interests of the people in our care, it is useful to consider the Five Principles of the Mental Capacity Act (DCA, 2007). These include: a presumption of capacity; supporting individuals to make their own decisions; recognising these may be 'unwise' decisions; when decisions are made on behalf of a person, they must be made in their best interests; and the least restrictive option should be chosen. Mental capacity is known to fluctuate, so should be assessed at each encounter. It is also worth noting that in cases where a person is detained under the Mental Health Act [1983], this takes precedence, so the MCA [2005] doesn't authorise anyone to give the person treatment for mental disorder (DCA, 2007). Activity 2.3 uses a consultation with Mrs Fiona Smith to allow you to apply some of these principles.

Activity 2.3   Critical thinking: assessing capacity to consent

According to her daughter, Mrs Smith has 'not been herself' over the past week or so. She thinks the pain caused by her leg wound or perhaps the move away from her home of 50 years has caused a bit of confusion. You visit Mrs Smith as requested to assess her with the assumption she has mental capacity to consent to this. However, she appears confused as to where she is, although allows you to check her blood pressure, temperature and lower leg wound.

1. How might you assess her capacity to consent?
2. What would your priorities be?

Some example answers are provided at the end of the chapter.

Activity 2.3 asked you to apply the principles discussed around consent and mental capacity for an adult. The next section provides an outline of legal considerations when prescribing for children.

Consent and the Mental Capacity Act: children and young people

There are important legal principles around consent and capacity that apply specifically to children. The United Nations Convention on the Rights of the Child (1989) and the Family Law Reform Act [1969] defined a child as someone under the age of 18. The Children Act [1989] formalised the relationship between parent and child, defining parental responsibility, including being able to consent on their behalf. Parental responsibility is automatically conferred on the mother of the child, but only on the father if they were married at the time of the child's birth (Children Act [1989], section 2) or if subsequently married (Family Law Reform [1987], section 1). For the purposes of consent and prescribing (or medicines administration, such as vaccinations) it is important to note the various laws in place regarding automatic, acquired or delegated parental responsibility, as these are complex and vary between the four UK countries.

There are limits to parental responsibility in that some decisions cannot be made by one parent alone – for example, sterilisation, circumcision, or hotly disputed immunisation (Griffith and Tengnah, 2017). Parental responsibility can be overridden by a court as it has jurisdiction to act in the child's best interest. The Family Law Reform Act [1969] presumes that young people have the legal capacity to agree to surgical, medical or dental treatments and associated procedures (with some exceptions). When a young person with capacity agrees to treatment, their decision to consent must be respected (DCA, 2007). However, *difficult issues can arise if a young person has legal and mental capacity and refuses consent – especially if a person with parental responsibility wishes to give consent on the young person's behalf* (DCA, 2007, p221). When the child has capacity and agrees to treatment, this can override their parents' wishes, but when they refuse treatment and there is disagreement, the Family Division of the High Court can be involved.

Decision-making capacity for children and young people can be seen as three stages towards autonomy:

1. a child
2. a Gillick competent child and
3. young people 16 and 17 years old.

(Kennedy and Grubb, 1998)

A child who has been assessed as having the maturity and intelligence to consent to examination or treatment is considered to be 'Gillick competent' (Gillick v West Norfolk and Wisbech AHA [1986]). Although 'Gillick' does not apply in Scotland, children have a right to consent to treatment under the Age of Legal Capacity (Scotland) Act 1991. As legal capacity is linked to a child gradually developing maturity, it is *dependent on the gravity of the situation* and the significance of the decision being made (Griffith and Tengnah, 2017, p192). So, for instance, while a younger child may understand and consent to having a plaster applied, they may not have the intelligence, maturity or capacity to consent to a surgical procedure.

For those working with children 16–18 years, NICE (2018a) suggests that *decision-making and mental capacity can be a particularly complex area.* NICE (2018a) also reminds that if a young person over 16 is found to lack capacity to make a particular decision, it is important to follow the same Mental Capacity Act [2005] best interests process and involve young people in decisions made on their behalf. When it is not appropriate for someone with parental responsibility to make a decision on behalf of the young person who lacks capacity, the MCA Code of Practice (DCA, 2007) should be followed to determine who should lead the 'best interests' process. Activity 2.4 asks you to critically consider the legal implications of prescribing, supplying and administering medications for children.

Activity 2.4   Critical thinking

There are specific legal aspects to be familiar with when caring for children and young people, particularly around consent and capacity. Identify some of the situations whereby you will need to be aware of these.

An outline of possible answers can be found at the end of the chapter.

Now that we have discussed the broad legal aspects of duty of care, consent and capacity, the next section provides an outline of key legislation concerned with the prescription, supply and administration of medicines.

The legal basis of nurse prescribing

As introduced in Chapter 1, prescribing by nurses has developed over time from a series of reports (DoH, 1989, 1999 (commonly known as the first and second Crown reports)), health policies and their implementation in law. The main sources of legislation underpinning prescribing derive from Acts of Parliamentary (statute law) and secondary legislation (statutory instruments). There are other sources of primary legal materials, such as judicial decisions and European Community and Human Rights law. V300 nurse independent prescribers (denoted on the NMC register as V300) can legally prescribe any product from the BNF within their scope of practice with the exception of three specific controlled drugs for the purposes of addiction treatment (Human Medicines Regulations [2012], Misuse of Drugs Act Amendment [2012]). This authority to prescribe is underpinned by key legislation outlined in Table 2.1, and any subsequent amendments or other secondary legislation. There are different laws and/or policies covering prescribing in the four UK countries.

Initial legislation covering medicines, the Medicines Act [1968], pertained to doctors and dentists only. While it is not entirely repealed, many parts of it have been replaced

Primary UK legislation	Secondary UK legislation	
Medicines Act [1968] *(almost wholly repealed)*	Prescription Only Medicines (Human Use) Order 1997 (SI 1997/183)	The Human Medicines Regulations [2012]
	Medicines for Human Use (Prescribing) (Misc. Amendments) Order 2006 (SI 2006/915)	
Misuse of Drugs Act [1971]	Misuse of Drugs Regulations 2001 (SI 2001/3998)	The Misuse of Drugs (Amendment No.2) Regulations 2012
European Community Law		
Criteria for determining products which should be available on prescription only – Directive 92/26/EEC.		

Table 2.1 UK legislation

over the years through amendments and legislation such as statutory instruments. Most laws for nurse prescribing involved amendments to this original Act, along with changes to central healthcare policy across the UK countries. The initial legislation to enable nurses to prescribe in the UK is the Medicinal Products: Prescription by Nurses Act [1992] which amended the Medicines Act [1968] and the NHS Act [1977]. As is still the case for community practitioner nurse or midwife prescribers (denoted by V100 or V150), this legislation only permitted prescribing from the Nurse Prescribers' Formulary (NICE, NPAG), limited to a select number and type of products.

Further legislation followed over the years, each of which incrementally added to the legal authority to prescribe. Other legal changes impacted more widely on medicines management, such as for mixing drugs (in syringe drivers). The largest piece of new legislation was the Human Medicines Regulations [2012] that consolidated over 200 separate pieces of law, orders, regulations or European directives that had built up over the years, without fundamentally changing medicines law (Griffith, 2012). Areas covered by these regulations include: the definition and classification of medicinal products, oversight and administration of medicines law, licensing of medicines, herbal, homeopathic and unlicensed medicines, borderline products, medicines safety and *pharmaco-vigilance*, the sale, supply and administration of prescription-only medicines and authorised exemptions from the general law, patient group directions (PGDs) and patient specific directions (PSDs). While the focus of this text is on prescribing, it is also incumbent on nurses to be aware of the laws surrounding medicines management more broadly, including other sources of authority for the supply of medicines, such as PGDs and PSDs.

Legal definitions of prescribing, supply and administration of medicines

In addition to prescriptions, there are other mechanisms by which patients can legally receive medications. Prescribing was initially by doctors or dentists only and is most often done using a legally recognised prescription form (in primary care) which is slightly different in each of the four countries (FP10 in England, WP10 in Wales, GP10 in Scotland, HS21 in Northern Ireland) and can be colour coded for different types of prescribers or prescriptions (PSNC, 2019). NHS Digital (2019a) predicts that the electronic prescription service (EPS) used to transfer prescriptions electronically between GP practices and pharmacies will eventually remove the need for most paper versions. Hospitals normally record prescribing via the patient record, while internal hospital forms are used for recording outpatient prescriptions being dispensed in the hospital pharmacy. PSDs, PGDs, professional exemptions and the legal requirements of a safely written prescription are outlined.

Patient specific direction (PSD)

The Royal College of Nursing (2019a) define this as a *written instruction, signed by a prescriber for medicines to be supplied and/or administered to a named person after the prescriber has assessed the person on an individual basis.* While in day-to-day practice this may be referred to as a 'prescription' it is not the same as an FP10, etc. that is subject to Human Medicines Regulations [2012] or other written prescriptions given to a person for supply from a pharmacy or dispensary. While a PSD must be a 'written' record, as opposed to a verbal instruction, it can be by hand or electronically – for example, in the hospital setting, this can be an instruction written on an inpatient's medicine chart. The CQC (2019) states that a PSD can also be an instruction to administer a medicine to a list of named individuals, but unlike a PGD each person on the list must be individually assessed by that prescriber and a judgement made as to the suitability in relation to the person's health and the appropriateness of the medicine to be administered. The CQC (2019) state that inspections have revealed instances where staff have mistakenly believed they were administering/supplying a medicine with the authority of a PSD. The following are some examples that do not meet the requirements of a PSD and are therefore not a legal authority for the administration or supply of medicines:

- a patient group direction (PGD) template that has been renamed a 'PSD' and used to instruct healthcare staff;
- a generic instruction to be applied to any person who may be seen by a healthcare professional or who has an appointment on any particular day – for example, an instruction to administer a 'flu vaccine' to any person who fits the criteria attending clinics on a specific day;
- a verbal instruction.

Patient Group Direction (PGD)

PGDs allow specified practitioners to supply and/or administer a medicine without a prescription or an instruction from a prescriber (Cavanagh, 2020). The RCN (2019a) advises that although a PGD is not a form of prescribing, the same process of assessing the person receiving the treatment should be undertaken. PGDs differ from PSDs as they are agreed group protocols in the form of written instructions that allow specific medicines to be supplied or administered to people who may not be individually identified prior to presenting for treatment (NICE, 2017a). The supply or administration is at the discretion of an authorised, named practitioner from one of the professions who is legally permitted to work to the PGD (MHRA, 2017). The medicines can be supplied or administered after ascertaining the recipient fits the criteria set out in the PGD (Human Medicines Regulations [2012], Cavanagh, 2020).

The legal requirements for PGDs are noted in the Human Medicines Regulations [2012]. NICE (2017a) suggests they should be written by a multi-disciplinary group and agreed by an authorising body (such as NHS England). NICE (2017a) suggests limiting their use to situations where there is a clear advantage to healthcare and treatment cannot be supplied in other ways. As inferred by the process by which PGDs are authorised, a nurse prescriber cannot write a PGD, although they can use it to supply or administer if appropriate.

Exemptions from prescribing

The **MHRA** (2014) outlines three ways that medicines can be sold and supplied in the UK. These are:

- on a prescription referred to as prescription-only medicines (POMs);
- in a pharmacy without prescription, under the supervision of a pharmacist (P);
- as a general sale list (GSL) medicine and sold in general retail outlets without the supervision of a pharmacist.

The Human Medicines Regulations [2012] contains exceptions to the general rules on selling, supplying and/or administering medicines for some groups of healthcare professionals including podiatrists, midwives or paramedics. There are no exemptions for nurses, but midwives, for example, can administer specific POMs such as adrenaline, diamorphine or oxytocin (MHRA, 2014).

Prescribing controlled drugs, unlicensed or off-label medicines

Independent prescribers (V300) are legally permitted to prescribe most controlled drugs (with the exception of three specific drugs for addiction treatment). These prescriptions have more stringent requirements, mainly for safety purposes. For example, prescribers should not exceed a maximum quantity of 30 days' supply for controlled drugs. In the past, all CD prescriptions needed to be hand written, but now can be computer generated and should include 'CD' after the order: e.g. Codeine 30mg tablets CD.

Prior to changes in legislation, nurses or prescribers were not legally able to mix medications before administering (DoH, 2010). Bentley *et al.* (2015) suggest mixing medications always poses a risk due to potential incompatibility. Some examples include physicochemical reactions within the mixture that can cause precipitation, separation, etc., or chemical instability leading to reduced effectiveness of one or all of the active ingredients, etc. (Bentley *et al.*, 2015). An example incompatible combination is oxycodone and cyclizine in a syringe driver (BNF, JFC). While prescribers can now legally mix medications as appropriate, it is important to use caution. To minimise the risks, the DoH (2010) recommend:

- the mixing of medicines should
  - only be undertaken in the best interests of the person in receipt
  - be avoided where possible
  - only be done by a person competent and willing to do so
  - take place in a pharmacy, where possible;
- prescribers should *seek advice from a pharmacist in deciding whether there are alternatives to administering mixed medicines for individual patients* and in determining which substance(s) can be mixed and in what dosages and that unlicensed products should be avoided.

Independent prescribers (V300) are legally permitted to prescribe off-label and unlicensed medicines within their scope of practice (Human Medicines Regulations, [2012]). DoH (2010) defines these as *a medicine which does not have a valid Marketing Authorisation (licence) in the UK.* The GMC (2021) states that *unlicensed medicines are commonly used in some areas of medicine such as in paediatrics, psychiatry and palliative care,* where it could be seen as unethical to do the research required for licensing. The GMC (2021) advises those prescribing an unlicensed medicine must be satisfied that there is adequate evidence of its safety, take responsibility for the decision and care, and maintain accurate and legible record-keeping including reasons for prescribing an unlicensed medicine. They also suggest providing sufficient information to allow informed decision-making, although recognise in certain circumstances this could cause distress. Off-label or off-licence medicines do have a licence, but describe the use of licensed medicines in a dose, age group, or by a route not in the product specification. Only prescribers (V300) can prescribe off-label but in doing so take full responsibility and are accountable for any harm caused by off-licence prescribing or administration. Nurse prescribers (V100 / V150) <u>cannot</u> prescribe unlicensed products and the only exception for 'off-license' products is nystatin for neonates (PSNC, 2021).

The law requires that medicines are prescribed, dispensed and administered to a person safely. The five 'R's outline that medicines should be given to: the right person, at the right time, in the right form, using the correct dose, via the right route. To support this, another legal requirement in fulfilling a duty of care as a prescriber is that of clear hand writing. As harm may occur to people who have received an illegible prescription, there is a legal requirement for prescription writing to meet an acceptable standard. If care is initiated through a care plan and harm results because others could not read your writing then liability in negligence is likely to arise (Prendergast v Sam and Dee Ltd [1989]).

The legal requirements of a valid prescription

The BNF (NICE, JFC) outlines the minimum legal requirements and key features of a safe prescription. Prescriptions for controlled drugs have additional legal requirements and there is additional guidance in the BNF that helps to ensure safe prescription writing, such as limited the use of abbreviations.

The BNF states prescriptions must:

- be written legibly in ink or otherwise so as to be indelible;
- be dated;
- state the name and address of the patient;
- state the address of the prescriber;
- provide an indication of the type of prescriber;
- be signed in indelible ink by the prescriber;
- state the age and DOB for children under 12 years;
- state the current weight of the child (as appropriate).

Prescriptions should include:

- the age and the date of birth of the patient;
- the weight of the patient where it has been used for a dose calculation.

Medicines or product details should include:

- the drug or preparation *name*
  - not abbreviated
  - using approved titles only
  - generic unless a specific brand is required
  - avoiding generic titles for modified-release preparations;
- the drug/preparation *form* (e.g. capsules, tablets, lozenges, suspension);
- the *strength* or quantity to be contained in the product (e.g. 125 mg/5 mL);
- the *dose*;
- the *dose frequency*
  - in the case of preparations to be taken 'as required' a minimum dose interval should be specified
  - care should be taken to ensure children receive the correct dose of the active drug. Therefore, the dose should normally be stated in terms of the mass of the active drug (e.g. '125 mg three times daily');
- the *quantity to be supplied*
  - this may be stated by indicating the number of days of treatment required in the box provided on NHS forms
  - items 'as required': if the dose and frequency are not given then the quantity to be supplied needs to be stated

- o   the quantity can be added for any item for which the amount cannot be calculated;
- *directions*
  - o   should preferably be in English without abbreviation, but it is recognised that some Latin abbreviations are used (as denoted in the BNF).

It is advisable to access your own employers' prescribing policy on prescription requirements. For instance, there is currently no nationally agreed design for the medicine chart, which varies in format between different hospitals or organisations. For primary care prescriptions, local policy may provide guidance for writing 'directions for use' as these need to be evidence-based and clearly stated. The online BNF (NICE, JFC) provides additional information regarding computer-issued prescriptions.

This section provided an overview of some of the legal aspects of prescribing; in the following some of the ethical principles are explored.

Ethical issues and prescribing

Ethics is seen as 'moral philosophy' and involves considering the fundamental questions around what is right and wrong. Morals are so widely shared that they form a social consensus. We may not always share these views of wider society and need to be aware that our decisions are influenced consciously or unconsciously by our value system. Östman *et al.* (2019) describe ethics as universal rules of conduct that help guide our actions, intentions and motives. Looking at prescribing from an ethical perspective can help to inform our decision-making. Professional morality can be seen as behaviours which are commonly accepted by professionals as part of their responsibilities (Beauchamp and Childress, 2019) and outlined in professional codes of conduct.

As a health professional, ethical practice needs to be balanced with the underpinning professional principles and the legal aspects of practice. Awareness of these help individual practitioners and healthcare teams examine the consequences of clinical decisions, and unpick the often complex challenges of clinical practice. When making clinical decisions moral analysis can begin, for example, when there is confusion about competing alternatives for action; when values of the healthcare team and the values of the family are in conflict about what is in the best interest of a patient or when a true dilemma emerges in which none of the alternatives is entirely satisfactory.

Four core principles of biomedical ethics were identified by Beauchamp and Childress (2019) as relevant to healthcare settings:

- *beneficence*: obligation to provide benefits and to balance benefits against risks;
- *non-maleficence*: the obligation to avoid causing harm;
- *respect for autonomy*: the obligation to respect the decision-making capacities of autonomous persons;
- *justice*: obligations of fairness in the distribution of benefits and risks.

Vincer and Kaufman (2017) link these four principles to those of medicines optimisation. The example includes: the aim to understand the patient's experience (respect for autonomy); employ evidence-based medicine choices (beneficence); ensure medicines use is as safe as possible (non-maleficence); and make medicines optimisation part of routine practice (justice) (Vincer and Kaufman, 2017). Each of the principles is explained further below.

Beneficence

Beneficence is the principle of doing 'good' for people and is fundamental to practice and embedded in professional codes. However, it may not always be straightforward as it entails a balance between benefits and risks, as well as considering whose perception of 'good' is given more credence. For example, as a nurse prescriber you may be aware that the benefits of compression bandaging far outweigh the risks of discomfort or harm and, in terms of evidence-based practice, are aware it is considered the 'gold standard'. However, from the perspective of the person receiving care the discomfort may result in this treatment not being seen as beneficial. The risks, benefits, costs and the varying perspectives should be taken into account when identifying treatment options. With a growing emphasis on informed choice, 'doing good' may also relate to education and information giving.

Non-maleficence

This principle simply means the person receiving care is not harmed by the professional. However, as most treatments involve risk of harm, even if minimal, it is important that the harm is not disproportionate to the benefits of treatment. Clearly, some harm is unforeseen, but the principle guides our decision-making and may influence the level of risk we are willing to take. For example, if a particularly nasty side effect was witnessed by the prescriber, this could influence their choice of treatment in the future. It is an important part of prescribing to be self-aware of the influences of your previous experience.

In relation to informed choice, while information giving and advice is generally seen as beneficent, it may also need to be balanced with the person's mental state, how much they can understand or want to hear at that time. For example, a person could be in denial of their diagnosis of end-stage heart failure and information giving causes distress and anxiety. However, there may also be pressure to treat someone urgently to prevent deterioration and the risk of entering the final stages of heart failure. As a professional, you may be aware that a lack of treatment is likely to result in harm, so when someone refuses treatment, you may need to weigh up which course of action would result in the least harm. This may involve questions around what is in a person's 'best interest', which is both a legal term and an ethical principle.

Autonomy

It has been established in law that a person's autonomy is core. This refers to respecting the decision-making for people assessed as having mental capacity and enabling individuals as far as possible to make reasoned and informed choices. Respect for autonomy in healthcare settings includes the need to gain consent for assessment, examination and investigation(s), as well as treatment. Autonomy requires an active listening approach so that the person in your care has the opportunity to have their views and choices heard and taken into account. Autonomy can be partial – for example, if a person has been legally assessed as not having the mental capacity for certain treatment decisions. From an ethical perspective, the views of someone with compromised mental capacity should still be taken into account and respected as far as possible.

Justice

The principle of justice concerns distributing benefits, risks and costs fairly. It suggests that patients in similar positions should be treated in a similar manner with healthcare services and medications shared in an equitable, non-discriminating way. It may be relevant to consider cost effectiveness of the treatment options for individuals and the impact treatment decisions have on the availability of treatment for others. If one was to view the principle of 'justice' as extending to the recognised NICE guidelines and formularies, it could produce a conflict with beneficence or autonomy if the person's preferred choice isn't available due to the product being deemed too costly. Activity 2.5 presents a scenario for you to consider the four key ethical principles.

Activity 2.5   Critical thinking: antibiotic prescribing

Cath has rung up the NHS111 service and your practice assessor (a V300 prescriber) is the nurse on duty. Cath reports the symptoms of a mild urinary tract infection, which she has had in the past, and would like some antibiotics. Because Cath's mum has become more confused, she is unable to leave the house to get to the GP or a clinic and wants to pre-empt it getting any worse. You go through the checks including ones to rule out sepsis, and are trying to decide if it is ethical to prescribe when it might not be necessary; you have a duty in relation to antibiotic stewardship. Relate this scenario to the four ethical principles discussed.

Activity 2.5 looked at the four principles of biomedical ethics in relation to antibiotic prescribing. The next section explores the ethical theories of deontology and utilitarianism.

Deontology and utilitarianism

As touched upon in relation to the principle of justice, there can be opposing moral views on beneficence for the wider population as well as the individual. This question can be examined through considering deontology (doing one's duty) versus utilitarianism (doing the greatest good for the greatest number).

Deontology is based on rights and duty, and involves doing the right thing without regard to whether the end consequences are good or bad ('the means justifies the ends'). Utilitarianism is considered to be 'ends-based' and involves acting without regard to whether the way you achieve a good thing is right or wrong ('the ends justify the means').

A practical example of how these contrasting theories can be applied to prescribing is in considering NICE guidance. Best practice as well as an economic analysis to show the cost effectiveness of treatments is considered when developing guidelines (NICE, 2020a). NICE (2008, p4) defines cost effectiveness as *value for money; a specific healthcare treatment is said to be 'cost effective' if it gives a greater health gain than could be achieved by using the resources in other ways.* In this way, it can be seen as utilitarian as the purpose is to fairly distribute resources and enable the greatest number of people to be treated. This can come into conflict with doing your duty when a particular treatment or medicine is not approved in the guidelines, but is needed by the individual patient to whom you owe a duty of care. In relation to evidence-based practice, in Chapter 4 we further consider the development and place of guidelines, as well as adherence to and deviation from them.

Chapter summary

This chapter considered selected legal and ethical principles pertinent to prescribing practice. Some of the underpinning legislation concerning your accountability as a practitioner fulfilling your duty of care has been outlined. It is highlighted that a knowledge of the law is expected, and throughout the chapter it is implied that you need to be aware of limitations and only prescribe within your scope of practice.

Ethical questions can arise in everyday practice and as a prescriber, it is suggested you reflect on current practice and gain self-awareness of your personal and professional moral viewpoint. Evidence-based practice was mentioned in relation to meeting your duty of care, promoting autonomy and informed choice, and this will be explored further in Chapter 4. To fulfil professional, legal and ethical duties as a prescriber, expertise is needed in undertaking a person-centred, structured and thorough assessment of the people in your care. The next chapter considers assessment and structured consultation with people who may need a prescription.

Activities: suggested answers and discussion points

Answer to Activity 2.1 The four spheres of accountability

This scenario suggests a practitioner with relatively little experience, who may be expected to learn mainly through experience. Practitioners new to these types of situations may not always be fully aware of their limitations or that they could be working outside their scope of practice. Below are some suggested answers in that context.

- *Civil:* (litigation/negligence) Harm can occur from both acts and omissions. It is advised to develop expertise through both additional study and practice, particularly when working in areas where there is the likelihood of undifferentiated diagnoses or co-morbidities – for example, undertaking a course in asthma management, or diabetes, etc. The expectation is for your decisions to be evidence-based and you can provide a sound explanation for either adhering to or deviating from the recognised clinical guidelines.
- *Criminal:* While this is a less likely consequence, it is worth noting that doctors have been prosecuted in a criminal court and jailed for a number of reasons, including, for example, failing to diagnose diabetes.
- *Professional:* Whether you are referred to the NMC to assess fitness to practise depends on several factors, including (but not limited to): the severity and nature of the harm, if it were linked to your acts or omissions, if you were not following the professional Code in some way or if your employer or someone else refers you.
- *Employment:* As above, this depends if the contract of employment were breached.

Strategies to reduce the risk would be to be aware of learning needs, seek continuing professional development opportunities, identify a supervisor or mentor, follow organisational policy, raise concerns as indicated and speak up, seek assistance, or onward refer when you encounter responsibilities or situations outside your scope of practice.

Answer to Activity 2.2 Critical thinking: duty of care – informed choice

This question revolves around some of the challenges you may face when making prescribing decisions for individuals in your care. Because each person will be different in their clinical presentations, medical history, knowledge, experience, health beliefs and desired outcomes from the encounter, it is important to consider informed choice and barriers to this. Below are some suggested answers in that context.

- *Biomedical:* there may be physical difficulties with communication such as hearing or speech impairment. The condition presented can be unclear or difficult to diagnose, impacting on the treatment choices. It may also be that there is limited information about the condition or product(s) to be prescribed. While we aim to promote informed choice, it may be that there is little flexibility in the treatment choice. When there is little to choose from, it may be necessary to weigh up the risks and benefits of treatment versus no treatment.
- *Psycho-social:* (comprehension) there is an assumption that people in your care have the mental capacity to make decisions. The assumption of capacity is stated within the Mental Capacity Act (2005) and the onus is on practitioners to communicate in a suitable way. Some people may be assessed as lacking the capacity to understand benefits and risks or consent to treatment. While there is less scope to promote informed choice in these instances, prescribers are expected to promote autonomy as far as possible.
- *Psycho-social:* (anxiety or emotional distress) several factors can impact on a person's emotional state including pre-existing conditions, the nature of their problem, social support systems and what stage they are at when you encounter them. Part of your duty would be to be aware how much they grasping and if it is safe to postpone the treatment decision.

Answer to Activity 2.3 Critical thinking: assessing capacity to consent

In addition to the two-stage test for assessing capacity, the DCA (2007) suggests asking further questions when assessing ability to make a decision. It's also worth considering if a more thorough assessment (for example, by a doctor or other professional expert) is needed, particularly for more complex or serious decisions. In this case, a referral would likely be indicated if it is a new and undiagnosed condition.

Implied consent

Through assessment of the situation and Mrs Smith, you can ascertain her level of understanding, checking her ability to retain and repeat back information. The detail of explanation should be proportionate to the task – for example, simply gaining consent to take her blood pressure requires less detail than if you were advising a hospital admission. As the scenario suggests, Mrs Smith allowed blood pressure, etc. to be checked; this could be through 'implied consent'. Holding out her arm and rolling up her sleeve is enough to enable the practitioner to undertake the procedure and record this as consent being obtained.

Consent from others

As family members were present, it would be possible to record their support for consenting to assessment as acting in the best interest of Mrs S. It is also an argument that assessment is required to ensure there are no life-threatening risks, which is part of our duty of care.

Priorities

- As this 'impairment' is new, you would want to try to ascertain the details such as duration, severity, how different this is from her usual mental state, what has been done so far and who else might be involved in her care. It would also be important to rule out any red flag or urgent/serious reasons behind the change in mental state so as to measure the urgency of your onward referral.
- Using recognised tools, you would then assess her ability to understand the purpose of any investigations or treatments or referrals you need to undertake.
- Where procedures, investigations or treatment may cause distress, or involve formal consent like an operation, then a multi-disciplinary approach or the involvement of expert practitioners is indicated. More significant decisions aren't made in isolation and the support of colleagues should be sought.

See also: GMC (2018a) *Consent: Patients and Doctors Making Decisions Together.*

Activity 2.4 Critical thinking

1. *Assessing and treating a child*: any time you encounter someone who is younger than 18, you need to be aware of the legal aspects for assessing their capacity to consent to examination or treatment (see recommended reading). When assessing a child's ability to consent, Griffith (2013, p711) suggests the child's intelligence and maturity be evaluated in relation to a number of other factors, such as that there is a choice to be made and that choices have consequences, the nature and purpose of the procedure, risks, or consequences of no treatment, etc.

2. *Administering immunisations*: this can be an emotive issue with potential for differences of opinion between parents. It is crucial that you are aware of the laws around consent and parental responsibility before treating a 'child of tender years'. It is also important to have a grasp of Gillick competence for immunisation of young people who may have the maturity and intelligence to consent. When a child is deemed Gillick competent, the consent is *as effective as that of an adult* (Griffith and Tengnah, 2017, p192).

3. *Contraception*: while not covered in the main section, if you are likely to encounter young people who require contraception advice, supply or prescribing (including emergency contraception), you need to be fully aware of the legal requirements around assessing Gillick competence, as well as the Fraser guidelines.

Please see Further reading for some additional guidance.

Activity 2.5 Critical thinking: antibiotic prescribing

Beneficence: There are many obstacles to remote prescribing, including a lack of both visual cues and the inability to physically examine the patient (Burton Shepard, 2019). Due to these challenges, you would need to weigh up whether you had enough information to safely make a treatment decision and to arrive at a beneficial outcome.

Non-maleficence: As a priority is to cause no harm, the risks and benefits of remote prescribing should be assessed at every stage of the consultation in order to provide safe effective care (Burton Shepard, 2019). There is a greater risk of missed cues and the lack of testing – for example, if a urine dip was indicated.

Autonomy: Part of the advantage of remote prescribing is convenience for the person seeking healthcare. Being able to complete the episode of care could be seen as promoting autonomy. Further, it could be seen that Fiona is taking control of her situation by pre-empting a likely worsening event and, having previous experience, could be seen as having a degree of expertise.

Justice: It could be argued that remote prescribing has potential to add to the efficiency of the health service, thus distributing the time resources more evenly. However, the counter-argument is that this individual is not necessarily receiving an assessment and examination that is equivalent to a face-to-face encounter. An important question to prompt continual improvement of assessment, examination and diagnostic skills is to ask yourself if the people you are caring for have received a safe and fair level of service. A further point of justice relates to antimicrobial stewardship and the need to think of the bigger picture, so as to do the greatest good for greatest number of people (a principle of utilitarianism).

Further reading and useful websites

We explored the concept of duty of care, with less emphasis on the duty of candour. You may wish to read about the legal and professional duty further in this article:

Dalton, D and Williams, N (2014) Building a Culture of Candour: A Review of the Threshold for the Duty of Candour and of the Incentives for Care Organisations to be Candid. http://www.rcseng.ac.uk/policy/documents/CandourreviewFinal.pdf

As part of professional practice, there was a discussion of consent and capacity. It is advisable to be familiar with the Mental Capacity Act (2005) and its code of practice (DCA, 2007).

Linked to the MCA (2005) deprivation of liberty of liberty standards. https://www.gov.uk/government/publications/deprivation-of-liberty-safeguards-forms-and-guidance

Applying the principles of mental capacity to children involves Gillick competence and to a lesser extent, Fraser guidelines.

- Care Quality Commission (CQC) (2018) *Nigel's surgery 8: Gillick Competency and Fraser Guidelines.*
- General Medical Council (GMC) (2018b) *0–18 Guidance for All Doctors.*

We briefly discussed the Mental Health Act and that it is separate from the Mental Capacity Act. You may wish to read these documents which provide further explanation of the Act and its practical application.

Department of Health and Social Care (DHSC) (2015a) *Mental Health Act 1983: Code of Practice Presented to Parliament pursuant to section 118 of the Mental Health Act 1983.* https://www.gov.uk/government/publications/code-of-practice-mental-health-act-1983

Department of Health and Social Care (DHSC) (2015b) *Mental Health Act 1983: reference guide.* https://www.gov.uk/government/publications/mental-health-act-1983-reference-guide

The legal principles and precedents can be challenging to grasp. You may wish to read further about some of these on the Wikibooks website, keeping in mind the need to also find research-based information.

Wikibooks (2017) *English Tort Law/Introduction* [online]. The Free Textbook Project. https://en.wikibooks.org/w/index.php?title=English_Tort_Law/Introduction&oldid=3214995

Chapter 3

Assessment and consultation

Chapter aims

After reading this chapter, you will be able to:

- explore frameworks and models of consultation to contribute to skilled and effective assessment of people and their presenting clinical need;

(Continued)

(Continued)

- identify a strategy for systematically gathering and interpreting information to aid diagnosis and facilitate person-centred clinical decision-making;
- outline an approach to safe and effective information-giving for suggested treatment, advice, safety-netting, follow-up and monitoring.

Introduction

Scenario

You and your practice assessor (a district nurse) are visiting Mrs Gill for her routine diabetic review. She is caring for her four-year-old granddaughter (Kira) and asks you to look at the sore area on her face as she's worried it may be infected. Your practice assessor has a quick look and says she thinks it is probably impetigo, so advises that Kira should see her GP.

The scenario with Mrs Gill reminds us that every encounter with a person in your care (and sometimes those who aren't) results in a clinical decision. These can range from taking no action, to providing advice, to initiating a treatment plan including a prescription. In this case, a brief assessment is reasonable as long as the advice is sufficient since Kira wasn't the main recipient of care. However, if, for example, she went on to develop sepsis, being able to explain decisions and documenting these is important. The safety of your clinical judgement is dependent on the accuracy and attentiveness of your assessment. This chapter explores how frameworks can help structure consultations and guide clinical decisions for the people in your care.

The chapter addresses RPS (2021a) prescribing competencies around assessment. These embrace the principle of acting in the best interests of people and putting them first to facilitate informed choice. It starts with a brief explanation of clinical decision-making and person-centred approaches. The next section considers structuring assessments efficiently, yet comprehensively for formulating a diagnosis, establishing priorities and identifying appropriate actions. Models of consultation and a structured prescribing framework are then explored. The bio-psycho-social model of healthcare is discussed as a way to establish the person's view of their presenting problems (Dossey and Guzetta, 2005; Conforth, 2013; Gough, 2018). The chapter concludes with the introduction of a clinical assessment tool RAPID-CASE which has been adapted from the National Prescribing Centre (NPC) (1999a, b) seven principles of good prescribing and the RPS Competency Framework (2021a).

Clinical decision-making

Using effective communication, future prescribers need to employ a systematic approach to consult with and appropriately assess the people in their care. Clinical assessment and consultation aim to address a clinical problem and normally include diagnosis, treatment and/or advice. Clinical consultations always entail making a decision. Figure 3.1 outlines example decisions.

Assessment and consultation models

People in your care may be well or have minor illness, exacerbations of long-term conditions, or significant life-limiting or acute problems. A host of biomedical, social or psychological influences on health are also of significance. Prescribing is one possible resolution from a range of options available when making decisions as a skilled practitioner with the legal authority to prescribe. Assurance that you have made the right decision at that time derives primarily from the quality of the assessment in determining the person's unique circumstance and preferences with other influencing factors including: the availability of options/resources, evidence-based practice, guidelines, protocols, formularies and/or expert advice and adherence to or deviation from guidelines as appropriate. Figure 3.2 illustrates some of these many influences.

To be able to articulate reasons for your decision-making, it is important to examine consultations and assessments. Thinking about your current practice, Activity 3.1 asks you to consider a recent clinical consultation with regards to how it was structured.

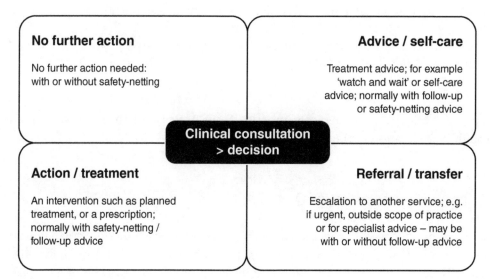

Figure 3.1 Clinical decision-making outcomes

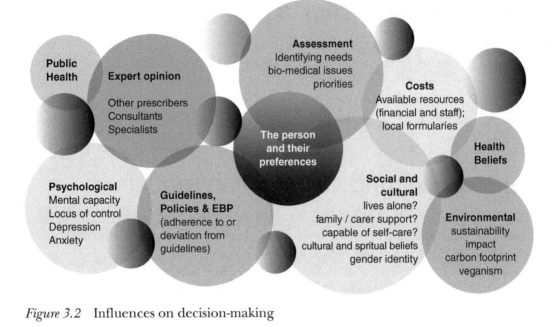

Figure 3.2 Influences on decision-making

Activity 3.1 Reflection

Consider a recent example from your practice, and the questions below. Asking these questions should enable you to reflect on whether you currently use a structured approach, and why you might want to do so.

- What was the presenting problem?
- How did you arrive at a decision?
- Was this a systematic process? If so, what model or structure was used?
- Why would you want to structure a clinical consultation/assessment?

As this activity is based on your own reflection there is no sample answer provided. It may help to observe your practice assessor and other experienced practitioners.

Keep your reflection on your own practice from Activity 3.1 in mind when reading through Jay's situation in the case study below.

Case study: Jay and Miss Q

Jay is a new prescriber who likes to take a thorough history when they prescribe. In clinic they see Miss Q who presents with the complaint of a longstanding leg ulcer, for which she self-cares. Jay undertakes the assessment following a known approach using a template, asking structured questions for about 20 minutes. From this Jay has gained what could be considered a full account of Miss Q's social, psychological and medical history. At the end of this time, however, Jay is still unsure what action to take, so asks Miss Q directly what she wanted from the consultation. Miss Q says she plans to continue with self-care but really just wants a repeat prescription for paracetamol as she has run out and it helps takes the edge off the leg pain.

As illustrated by the case study of Jay and Miss Q, alongside a structured approach it is essential to first establish the person's perspective and aim of their encounter with you as a health professional. Next, we look at a selection of assessment and consultation models to aid your clinical decision-making.

Assessment

People in your care are individuals with unique abilities, characteristics, preferences and needs. Assessments require us to ask the right questions, actively listen and make judgements, including attaching importance to or disregarding pieces of information. The word 'assessment' is historically related to judgement as 'assessors' were appointed to sit and decide cases alongside judges. This definition can be seen as relevant as the expectation is that you appraise, rate, or weigh-up information to make decisions, effect a plan and evaluate its impact as part of the nursing process. Emphasis on assessment allows you to individualise care, while frameworks or nursing models are used to put this problem-solving approach into practice. Identifying problems and priorities requires information collection through tools such as the 'activities of daily living' (Roper *et al.*, 2000). However, tools acting as set criteria for which assessment data are collected can be prescriptive and potentially limit a partnership approach as it is seen as the professional's role to determine a person's needs and priorities (Gough, 2018). If we want to practise in a person-centred way it is essential that the person's values are central in decision-making (McCance *et al.*, 2021).

Assessment can also be thought of as describing a variety of factors you need to know about a person. These include knowing the person, what their needs are now and might be in the future, what resources are available and what your own knowledge deficits are (Kennedy, 2004). This also reminds you to recognise limitations and work within your scope of practice (NMC, 2018a). Structured frameworks can enhance assessment with potential to improve patient care and outcomes (Munroe *et al.*, 2013). Conversely, poor assessment can be linked to delays in care, treatment or referral, misdiagnosis, error, harm, delays in recovery from the problem, or the absence of a baseline against which to judge the improvement or deterioration. Reflection on clinical assessment and consultation in current practice is a good way to develop your knowledge and skills. Activity 3.2 works through an example of this.

> ## Activity 3.2 Reflection
>
> Consider an example of an assessment you or your practice assessor carried out in practice and reflect on your awareness of how you structured this and how it 'flowed' or progressed. For example, was there a clear introduction that set out your aims for the encounter and gained the person's view of the aims? Was it conversational or did it follow a fixed template that limited open-ended questions? Was there a need to go back to missed questions or information? Now consider: if the same encounter was expected to result in issuing a prescription, would the assessment need to be different? Would further information need to be sought? Would the model, template or framework you currently use adequately address the points required to make a prescribing decision?
>
> *As this activity is based on your own reflection there is no sample answer provided. You may wish to discuss it with your practice supervisor.*

Keep your reflection on your own practice from Activity 3.2 in mind when reading through the sections on structured consultation.

Consultation

For the purposes of a prescribing decision a more methodical approach to assessment and its supporting documentation is advised to avoid missed information, premature closure and errors. In contrast to assessment definitions, consultation implies a more collaborative approach, being described as a meeting, discussion or appointment, normally with an expert or professional. Research undertaken many years ago, found that nurses in all clinical settings demonstrated problems with the organisation of their consultations (Hastings and Redsall, 2006b). For example, records available prior to the consultation weren't used effectively, and diagnostic tests or physical examinations were done before the person's information was obtained or considered. Hastings and Redsall (2006b, p12) observed a *notable tendency to move prematurely to care planning* before clearly identifying the key issue(s), ultimately making the consultations longer. Even if the range of conditions you encounter is narrow, structuring these by applying a consultation model is more efficient and better supports the clinical decision-making process (Hastings and Redsall, 2006b). Although not a model, the RPS (2021a) CFAP highlights a structured approach to consultation.

Structure is essential as you need to be able to explain how a decision was made, and what information underpinned the decision. In tandem with this is the need to establish the person's view of their problem(s) and the relative weight or priority they place on this. Other considerations include assessment templates you may be required to work with, time resource, the setting of the assessment and the mental capacity of those you are assessing, as these can all add complexity.

Baking a cake: the benefits of a recipe or consultation model

Consider the non-clinical example of baking a cake. You would normally follow a recipe and use a defined set of ingredients, although there is some flexibility depending on personal taste. You may make an excellent cake and share it with your colleagues who want to replicate it. This could be difficult, or even flawed without a recipe to explain how to progress through the stages of putting the ingredients together. While this may not always be a problem, the need for a clear explanation can arise if, for example, the cake failed or someone became ill afterwards.

In the clinical context, consultation models can be seen as the recipe, with assessment frameworks' discrete pieces of information as the ingredients or the key components. Like using a recipe to bake a cake, applying a structured approach with a consultation model will provide benefits to your practice including:

- enabling a clear starting point and conclusion;
- helping to keep within a timeframe (and meet the demands of a busy environment);
- limiting how many issues can be spoken about;
- assisting with moving the consultation forward;
- facilitating assurance that pertinent information has been attained;
- aiding consistency across different practitioner/assessors.

Consultation models

There are numerous 'medical' consultation models; more recent 'nursing' models have also been developed. These models aim to focus the assessment of people presenting with particular problems for which you are expected to make a clinical decision. Carter (2018) suggests consultation models are not rules, but instead *learning aids to help you develop your own consultation skills*. A number of common models are outlined below. These should be seen as the 'recipe' by which you undertake and progress the encounter, while adding specific questions or investigations as appropriate, as framed by a more detailed assessment tool. For example, using the Neighbour (1987) model, there are five steps describing how your consultation progresses. However, each of these can be seen as broad stages with specific questions or topics required. These specifics are discussed later in the chapter in relation to the 'RAPID-CASE' assessment tool.

No matter what tool or model you select, or in what context, it is fundamental that at every stage of encounters with people in your care you consider if the situation is urgent, or is likely to become urgent, or if it is outside your scope of practice, requiring advice or referral. A simple model to guide referral, triage and prioritisation is the 'traffic light system' (Red, Amber and Green).

> ## Concept summary: prioritisation
>
> This aims to help you identify when you need to:
>
> - *Stop (Red)*: Stop what you are doing and take urgent action. This is when what you are presented with requires immediate action, treatment or care, or referral is urgently needed.
> - *Proceed with caution (Amber)*: Further assessment required with possibility of referral. This is for when symptoms are not currently urgent, but they risk becoming urgent so action and/or safety-netting are required *within a specified time.*
> - *Continue (Green)*: Stable or routine. This is for when treatment or advice remains within your scope of practice, or referral does not need to be within a specified time. Symptoms need addressing and a plan putting in place, but it is within your scope of practice at this time to provide treatment, advice or onward referral.

As a prescriber, there will be more situations in which you have the autonomy and authority to conclude a complete episode of care without referral to other services or practitioners. A structured or rational approach to your decisions makes it easier to provide a clear explanation or rationale. Five example consultation models are presented below which were either originally identified by medical practitioners or psychologists, or have arisen since the advent of prescribing beyond the medical profession. The models tend to describe a series of stopping points along a timeline for your encounter with people when making a clinical decision. While reading through these different models, consider which is most appropriate for your area of practice.

Model 1: Pendleton et al. (1984)

This model concentrates on the patients' ideas, expectations and concerns (ICE). Harper and Ajao (2013) suggest it is a collaborative process which can also help with building the longer-term relationship. The steps aim to use a person-centred approach and the seven tasks are to:

1. define the reason why they are attending or seeking help;

2. provide consideration for other problems;

3. enable the person to choose an appropriate action for each problem;

4. come to a shared understanding of the problem;

5. involve the person to encourage their acceptance of responsibility and enable them to manage the problem;

6. use the time resources effectively and appropriately;

7. establish and keep a good relationship so that all these tasks and a good outcome can be achieved.

Model 2: Neighbour (1987)

This model describes the consultation as a journey with 'checkpoints' along the way. It includes stages to undertake with the person being assessed as well as attention to the need for the practitioner to reflect on and learn from the encounter. A good way to remember this is to use your hand and the different fingers for each checkpoint.

- *Checkpoint 1: CONNECTING* Has rapport with the person been developed?
- *Checkpoint 2: SUMMARISING* Why was the person seeking help? What were their expectations? Listening and examining as needed are part of this stage.
- *Checkpoint 3: HANDOVER* Has a shared understanding been reached? Is there a mutually acceptable plan?
- *Checkpoint 4: SAFETY-NETTING* This involves predicting how things may go and asking 'what if …?'. Advice regarding actions to take if problem persists, worsens or if a new problem occurs should be provided and the person's understanding of this checked.
- *Checkpoint 5: HOUSEKEEPING* This is when you reflect on how you are feeling after the encounter, and considering if you are able to move on to the next patient. This can include identifying areas where further information or professional skills or knowledge development is needed.

Model 3: Calgary–Cambridge guide to the medical interview (Silverman et al.,1998)

This model was developed by medical doctors to aid effective communication skills and to provide an evidence-based structure for their analysis and teaching. It takes a logical

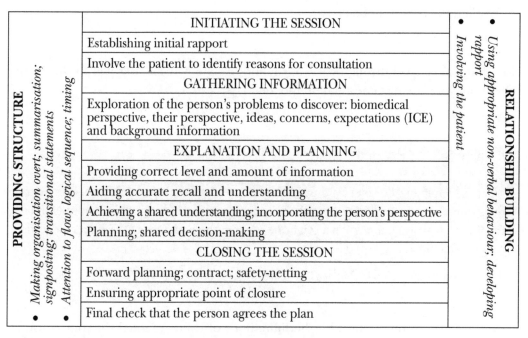

Table 3.1 The Calgary–Cambridge consultation model

sequence to the consultation from initiating the session, gathering information, giving information by explanation and planning, and closing the session. Supporting this is the need to provide clear structure to the consultation and build a relationship.

Model 4: A model of consultation (Hastings and Redsall, 2006b)

Hastings and Redsall (2006b) undertook research into nurse consultations when prescribing was not yet fully established so there was some resistance to the idea that nurses could make a diagnosis. Their observation that the structure of consultations needed a more logical sequence led to the development of their ten-point consultation model. This was alongside the Consultation Assessment and Improvement Instrument for Nurses (CAIIN), providing a useful method of peer or self-assessment.

1. Interpret prior knowledge about the person (e.g. through care records).
2. Set goals for the consultation.
3. Gather sufficient information to make a provisional 'triple diagnosis'.
4. Discover the person's ideas, concerns and expectations about the problem(s) (ICE).
5. Carry out appropriate physical examination and near-patient tests to confirm or refute the diagnosis.
6. Reconsider your assessment of the problem.
7. Reach a shared understanding of the problem with the person.
8. Give the patient advice about what they need to do to tackle the problem.
9. Explain the actions to be taken.
10. Summarise and close.

Now that you've read through each of the models, Activity 3.3 asks you to think critically about your use of a consultation model.

Activity 3.3   Critical thinking

What model, if any, do you currently use when consulting with people? If you don't currently use a model, which of those outlined above would you consider to be most useful for framing your consultations? What might be some of the limitations of using a model for your consultations?

An outline of possible answers about the limitations of models can be found at the end of the chapter.

Activity 3.3 asked you to consider the limitations of using a model for your consultations; this is now something we'll consider in more detail.

Limitations of using models

It has been recognised in the past that without the use of a model nurses tended to move too quickly to diagnosis and planning stage with the risk of missing important information or working inefficiently. However, it should also be noted that working within a framework or model can be a restriction, particularly if it involves the mechanical following of an assessment template without actively listening.

The importance of history-taking

As you can see from the example consultation models above, gaining the person's perspective and taking a thorough history is integral to the process of making a diagnosis. Any well-structured approach includes thorough history-taking. Older research into medical consultations found that history-taking *alone* produced over 80 per cent of accurate diagnoses, with relatively few (18 per cent) being changed after clinical investigations or physical examination (Hampton *et al.*,1975). Further to this, Peterson *et al.* (1992) found that despite advances in medical science, most diagnoses continue to be made from the medical history (Figure 3.3 below). Laboratory findings and physical examination are identified as important for excluding some diagnoses and help increase the practitioners' self-confidence in their diagnostic ability.

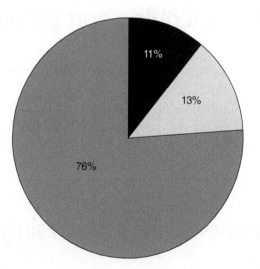

Figure 3.3 Diagnosis: history-taking; physical examination and investigations

(based on Peterson *et al.*, 1992)

We have considered some context for using a structured approach to assessment and consultation, with the exploration of some of the common models. It is suggested that a model is selected in line with personal preference and the context of the situation as a broad basis for the route the consultation takes. The models outlined thus far have been more generic for encounters with people requiring care rather than specifically for prescribing situations. We will now move on to focusing specifically on a consultation/assessment framework to aid prescribing decisions.

> RAPID-CASE is a new model to aid prescribing decisions that integrates features from consultation models, the original 'prescribing pyramid' (NPC, 1999b) and the Competency Framework for All Prescribers (RPS, 2021a).

RAPID assessment and CASE

As all encounters with people in your care lead to a clinical decision, it is important to be able to articulate why you have taken no action, given advice, onward referred, established a diagnosis, prescribed, or initiated a treatment plan. RAPID-CASE is a model for prescribing decisions that combines elements from consultation models, the 'prescribing pyramid' (NPC, 1999b) and the Competency Framework for All Prescribers (RPS, 2021a). The aim is to illustrate a structured approach that retains person-centredness while reminding you of specific information needed to make a safe prescribing decision. Within this model, the acronym RAPID is used for the clinical assessment, while CASE guides the choice of product(s).

The steps to prescribing competence

The prescribing steps introduced in Chapter 1 illustrate the full range of prescribing-related competencies (RPS, 2021a). Governance forms the foundation and needs to be embedded before and after your consultations. RAPID-CASE takes you to Step 4 of the competencies, so Step 5 and 6 would still be required, along with some of the governance items such as providing information, monitoring, reviewing and documentation to complete the episode, followed by reflecting on your prescribing.

RAPID-CASE model for prescribing assessment

The RAPID assessment tool in Figure 3.4 can be used to provide a structured consultation for decision-making in the prescribing context. Alongside this, the acronym CASE is used to outline considerations for making a case for the choice of product, medicine, prescribed treatment, de-prescribing or no treatment. This refers to the specific assessment to inform your decision and reminds of the aspects needed for safe and effective decision-making.

R	A	P	I	D
Rapport	**Assessment (bio-medical)**	**Psycho-social**	**Investigations**	**Diagnosis**
Consent/capacity Person's view of the health issue (presenting complaint – PC) Ideas, concerns, expectations	History of PC & actions so far Medical history Current health Allergy Status Medications	Social history Family history Social and mental well-being Potential vulnerabilities	Physical examination Tests Investigations Referral	Differential & Working diagnoses Summary Shared understanding

STOP AND THINK BEFORE PRESCRIBING — Is a prescription needed?	C	A	S	E
	Cost-effective	**Appropriate**	**Safe**	**Effective**
Self-care / Advice Referral Medicines Optimisation & De-prescribing	On formulary? Available OTC? Generic? Pack size?	Suitable for the person? Acceptable? Is concordance likely?	Contra-indications? Side-effects? Interactions? Safety-netting?	Evidence-based? Guidelines? Justifiable?

Figure 3.4   RAPID-CASE consultation model for prescribing

Structuring your consultation using the RAPID model

We'll now work through how you can use this model to structure your consultation.

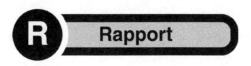

Rapport/initial stages

The first stage of RAPID is the rapport stage (see Figure 3.4) which starts prior to the consultation where you access and gather pertinent information from health records (as available). At the start of the consultation, you make introductions and begin to develop rapport. While this is usually through open questions, you will need to gain basic information such as checking identification (using name, address and date of birth (DOB)) and ensure a match with records you are using. If it is a remote (telephone or video) consultation, identify who you are speaking with – for example, is it the person themselves, or a carer, relative or parent. You also need to gain consent and assess the mental capacity of the person. Further to this, you can start to explore the person's own view of their health issue(s) using open questions, as well as how they may or may not have addressed it so far. Part of this conversation is establishing their priorities, for example by using *ideas, concerns and expectations* (ICE), as explored in Activity 3.4.

Activity 3.4 Reflection

The ICE acronym (ideas, concerns and expectations) can be used to understand the person's perspective and clarify their expectations. Reflect on a recent encounter in practice and consider if you would be able to describe a clear picture of the person's ideas, concerns and expectations. Further explanation of this model is included below to help you think this through.

I – Ideas: This involves asking open questions that help to illustrate their understanding of the health problem(s). For example, asking them to tell you a little bit about what has been happening, or why they are taking certain medications (as appropriate). They may be very knowledgeable or there can be a need to offer clarity or advice about the health condition or current treatment.

C – Concerns: This provides another opportunity to ascertain the person's main concerns, as these may be different to the information provided to you or your understanding of their presenting problem.

E – Expectations: This is where you would ask what they see as the likely or desired outcome. It is very useful to establish what they hope to gain through this encounter with you as a health professional.

As this activity is based on your own reflection there is no sample answer provided at the end of the chapter.

Activity 3.4 took you into more detail of the rapport stage, now we'll consider each of the other stages of this model in turn.

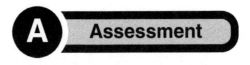

Assessment of biomedical

This stage is about getting the details and history of the presenting complaint, which may entail additional assessments such as a pain scale. Alongside this you will need to confirm the person's full medical history, any other current conditions, their allergy status, medication history including over the counter (OTC) or purchased medications, as well as any illicit drugs, alternative or herbal remedies, alcohol intake and smoking habits. It is also necessary to review their adherence to and the effectiveness of current treatment regimes, including medicines. With so much to remember at this stage, different acronyms may help, such as SOCRATES (Figure 3.5) for assessing pain, or JAM THREADS (Figure 3.6) that reminds of a variety of medical conditions.

The first of these, SOCRATES (Figure 3.5), is widely used to assess pain.

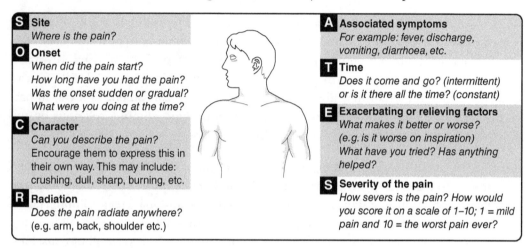

S Site	**A** Associated symptoms
Where is the pain?	*For example: fever, discharge, vomiting, diarrhoea, etc.*
O Onset	**T** Time
When did the pain start? *How long have you had the pain?* *Was the onset sudden or gradual?* *What were you doing at the time?*	*Does it come and go? (intermittent) or is it there all the time? (constant)*
C Character	**E** Exacerbating or relieving factors
Can you describe the pain? *Encourage them to express this in their own way. This may include: crushing, dull, sharp, burning, etc.*	*What makes it better or worse? (e.g. is it worse on inspiration) What have you tried? Has anything helped?*
R Radiation	**S** Severity of the pain
Does the pain radiate anywhere? (e.g. arm, back, shoulder etc.)	*How severs is the pain? How would you score it on a scale of 1–10; 1 = mild pain and 10 = the worst pain ever?*

Figure 3.5 SOCRATES

Understanding someone's medical history as well as any current conditions is a key part of this stage. The acronym JAM THREADS (Figure 3.6) can be used to remind you of a range of conditions that may affect your prescribing decision and gain information regarding their past medical history. There are other conditions not listed here, so remember to ask open questions about a person's medical history in addition to accessing records (where possible).

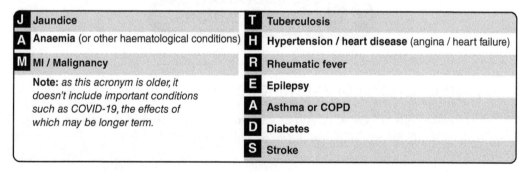

J Jaundice	**T** Tuberculosis
A Anaemia (or other haematological conditions)	**H** Hypertension / heart disease (angina / heart failure)
M MI / Malignancy	**R** Rheumatic fever
Note: *as this acronym is older, it doesn't include important conditions such as COVID-19, the effects of which may be longer term.*	**E** Epilepsy
	A Asthma or COPD
	D Diabetes
	S Stroke

Figure 3.6 JAM THREADS

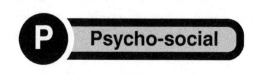

P Psycho-social

Psycho-social and context

For these aspects, a conversational approach may help to identify what is happening in the person's life and how this may be impacting on their view of the presenting issue(s). *Family history* involves ascertaining if there are any medical concerns of immediate family members (parents, sisters, brothers), which may have an impact on their current health or condition(s), such as heart disease or inherited conditions.

When considering their *social situation*, you would want to ask if they are working or retired and, as appropriate, can ask about living arrangements (e.g. if homeless, this may impact on treatment choices); their close relationships (e.g. married, divorced, etc.); if sexually active (as appropriate, e.g. presenting with signs of UTI). Health beliefs and health literacy may also form part of the social assessment as it can impact on disclosure of information or consent to treatment. For example, religious or cultural beliefs have been shown to affect uptake of vaccines.

Assessing a person's *mental wellbeing* is crucial. Assessment of mental capacity is needed for consent to assess or provide treatment. You will also want to know about any past psychiatric history; mood; signs of depression or anxiety; and may need to undertake a 'mini' mental health assessment using a recognised tool (such as those recommended by NICE – e.g. Whooley questions; depression and anxiety score) or level of consciousness as appropriate. The RPS (2021a) CFAP also mentions assessing for *vulnerabilities* that may be prompting the person to seek treatment or support. This can refer to psychological distress or safeguarding concerns which practitioners must always be alert to. For example, unexplained increases in prescribed drug use could be due to a person experiencing coercive control or abuse obtaining prescriptions for other people (drug diversion).

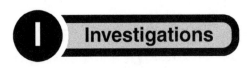

Investigations/clinical examination(s)

While history-taking prompts most diagnoses, examinations and investigations can be indicated to confirm or refute the working and differential diagnoses.

Physical examination

Depending on the situation, you may need to do a full 'head to toe' assessment/physical examination, or more specific clinical examinations. These should be undertaken as appropriate within your scope of practice. Medical doctors have been educated to be proficient at full physical examinations and advanced care practitioners should also have undertaken education to aid their ability to undertake fully physical examination.

Community formulary prescribers may not have studied advanced examination but require physical assessment skills, including specific ones such as for ear or wound examination, or digital rectal examination for constipation. Cathala and Moorley (2020) outline an 'A to G' assessment originally devised for emergency situations, but suitable for anyone receiving care. Examination of visible signs such as pallor, cyanosis, use of auxiliary muscles for breathing, skin conditions, redness, inflammation, wounds, etc. are important in everyday practice but for remote consultations skilled questioning is needed. Other signs such as smell or capillary refill also require additional questions, while it is still possible to listen out for signs of respiratory issues such as shortness of breath, coughing or wheezing.

When assessing for either local symptoms (such as rashes) or systemic signs (such as pallor), variations in natural skin tones should be considered. NICE (2015a) pressure ulcer guidance indicates that *non-blanchable erythema* may present differently in darker skin tones or types. Black and Simende (2020) suggest strategies for assessing darkly pigmented skin as there is a greater risk of higher-stage pressure injuries (Gunowa *et al.*, 2018). More generally, Rayner *et al.* (2021) advocate for midwives being 'colour aware' as opposed to being 'colour blind' due to the importance of skin examination for physical assessment of maternal and neonatal wellbeing. Mukwende *et al.* (2020) highlight a need for awareness of how symptoms and signs can present differently on darker skin as well as the need to adjust language used for descriptors.

Test and investigations

As per the physical examination, requests for investigations and tests should be done within your scope of practice, or onward referred as needed. Simple near-patient testing for urine or BM level can help aid diagnosis. For example, assessing a person whose wound is unexpectedly not healing may involve undertaking a BM to check for undiagnosed diabetes, prior to referring or requesting fasting blood sugars. Wound swabs are commonly used to identify colonisation or infection.

Results and findings

These can be used (as available) to confirm or exclude a working diagnosis. An understanding of normal values and the implications of deviations from these is an important way to confirm or rule out specific diagnoses or raise your alert to the need for referral.

Identifying red flag symptoms

Whether prescribing or not, it is important to be aware of symptoms that may be indicative of serious underlying issues and when to refer to or seek guidance from others. Red flags and causes for urgent referral cover a range of clinical problems. For example, nurse prescribers can issue nystatin for oral thrush, but there are potential 'red flag' symptoms for mouth ulcers or persistent oral thrush. Activity 3.5 explores this further, asking you to identify some red flag symptoms.

Activity 3.5   Critical thinking: evidence-based practice and research

Identify 2 or 3 'red flag' symptoms and outline the actions you would take for each of these.

For further information about red flags take a look at the resources below.

GP online resource. This provides quick summaries of alert signs and symptoms that indicate a more serious underlying pathology. Each article provides a list of red flags, possible causes and advice on history-taking and examination during the consultation and when to refer. See: https://www.gponline.com/education/medical-red-flags

NICE guidance on suspected cancer symptoms. Signs that may indicate cancer are outlined in the NICE guideline (NICE, 2017c). https://www.nice.org.uk/guidance/ng12

A sample answer is provided at the end of the chapter.

Activity 3.5 asked you to find some example red flag symptoms or reasons for urgent referral. Now we will consider the final stage of the RAPID model, making a diagnosis.

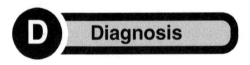

Diagnosis: working and differential diagnosis

While there was initially some debate over the use of the word 'diagnosis' for the activity of nurse prescribing, it is acknowledged that in order to initiate or prescribe treatment, the process by which this is safely done implies making a diagnosis. This involves gathering information and matching the findings or symptoms with the usual clinical picture. Similar to treatment decisions, diagnosing involves applying evidence and guidelines. Confirming the final diagnosis requires systematic consideration of the various possibilities (differential diagnoses). Activity 3.6 explores this process in a practical example.

> ## Activity 3.6 Decision-making: making a diagnosis – itchy scalp
>
> Sam is a four-year-old child who presents with a complaint of itchy scalp. You establish this has been for approximately two weeks and it is worsening. From the social and family history, you find she has an older school-aged sister who was recently treated for head lice. The mum reports there has been a notice about head lice at school. You ask about any family history of eczema and check for 'cradle cap'.
>
> - What is your working diagnosis?
> - What are your differential diagnoses?
> - What clinical signs would enable you to make a diagnosis?
>
> *A sample answer is provided at the end of the chapter*

Making a CASE for treatment decisions

Once the diagnosis is established as far as possible, as in Activity 3.6, the next steps involve determining the best course of action. While CASE is explored further in the next chapter on evidence-informed decision-making, it is introduced here as part of the prescribing steps. Embedded within it are RPS (2021a) competencies – for example, a shared understanding, agreeing a treatment plan and providing information (including safety-netting advice). Outcomes of decision-making other than a prescription such as de-prescribing or non-pharmacological alternatives should always be considered first.

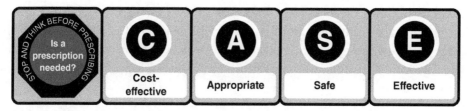

Figure 3.7 CASE

CASE

Once a decision to prescribe has been made (as opposed to referring onwards, offering advice, de-prescribing, non-pharmacological or alternative treatments), CASE refers to asking if the product to be prescribed is cost effective, appropriate, safe and effective.

> *Cost effective.* While cost effectiveness isn't necessarily the first consideration, if a medicine or product isn't available because of its cost, that affects your ability to

prescribe it. A part of our professional and moral duty is to be cost-aware and be able to justify our decisions. The local policies or formularies from which we select a product take cost into consideration.

Appropriate. This is where you use information gained from history-taking to check if the product is suitable for the individual. For example, whether they have any known allergies, or are taking anything that may cause potential **drug interactions**, or any cautions from pre-existing medical conditions. Certain groups of people require greater caution – for example, those at the extremes of age, or with liver or renal impairment. Along with the right product, the dose, formulation and the duration of treatment should be specific to the individual.

Safe. In addition to the cautions that are person-specific, medications hold some risk of harm so should be prescribed cautiously. Professionals need to keep abreast of 'alerts' and sign up to the regular service for these. If an adverse effect is suspected, it may need to be escalated and, if confirmed, should be reported through the Yellow Card system and noted on the person's medical record as appropriate.

Effective. Alongside the safety of a product, the prescriber needs to know which treatments are most effective. As a prescriber, you will be expected to have knowledge of recommended treatments, and to continually update this. The range of information sources will be discussed further in the next chapter. An excellent source to start with is the British National Formulary (BNF).

Shared understanding

Using RAPID-CASE will take you through most practical steps of the prescribing cycle, but this is to emphasise the importance of developing a shared understanding of the issues and the best way to address them. One of the stages to undertake before agreeing a treatment plan or prescribing is to check the shared understanding of the presenting problem and diagnosis at which you have arrived. This is normally done through summarisation and allowing opportunity for any other issues to be raised.

Prescribe: agreed treatment plan and/or advice

Following on from a shared understanding of the issue(s), the treatment plan, including any prescribed products and their use, needs to be agreed. This also includes any self-care advice, recommendations for over the counter or alternative products, decisions to de-prescribe, or for no treatment to be started at this time. Part of the responsibility for the treatment plan is to agree follow-up, monitoring and to provide clear safety-netting advice.

Provide information: safety-netting

This is where you assure that the person knows how to and when to seek advice. This can be in relation to a treatment you have initiated, the persistence or worsening of symptoms, or the development of new complaints. Safety-netting should include ascertaining the person's understanding of: when to seek help if the problem persists; what symptoms they should look for if the condition or problem worsens; what additional or new issues they should be alert to (for example, allergic or other adverse reactions to treatment); who to contact/where to seek advice or help; what would be considered urgent or an emergency.

Prescribing governance

Several aspects of the governance competencies are of pertinence at the end of the consultation, including the need for documentation and clear communication with others in the team. These concepts are explored in other chapters within the textbook.

Chapter summary

This chapter introduced the use of a structured approach to the assessment of an individual for the purposes of making a clinical decision. Throughout the chapter working within your scope of practice is emphasised as it is imperative to have the required level of skills and competence. A structured approach is recommended, using a consultation model for your encounters with people who may or may not need a prescription. A new model to aid prescribing decisions, RAPID-CASE, was introduced, highlighting that a systematic assessment is required to ensure your future prescribing is safe, effective, appropriate and cost effective. This is best achieved through person-centred communication that includes a mix of open and closed questions as you proceed through the consultation. Working in an evidence-based way was touched upon and will be explored thoroughly in the next chapter.

Activities: suggested answers and discussion points
Answer to Activity 3.3 Critical thinking

Sticking to a rigid model may:

- actively alter the persons' behaviour or responses;
- inhibit the disclosure of information;
- prevent equal participation within the consultation. A perceived imbalance of power may lessen partnership or inhibit the person from expressing their priorities;
- reduce shared decision-making, prevent a person-centred approach;
- result in missed cues or key information.

Answer to Activity 3.5 Critical thinking: evidence-based practice and research

There are many red flag symptoms and it is worth checking the resources regularly so you build up knowledge of a good range of these. A couple of more common examples are listed:

- **absence of peripheral pulses**: *due to the risk of ischaemia, gangrene, leading to amputation;*
- **constipation**: *change in bowel habit for more than six weeks, persistent rectal bleeding, weight loss, night sweats, appetite loss, family history of colorectal pathology, bowel distension, pain and vomiting, abdominal bloating, new-onset confusion, significant weight gain – these are red flags for bowel cancer but have many other possible causes.*

Answer to Activity 3.6 Decision-making: making a diagnosis – itchy scalp

- **What is your working diagnosis?** Head lice.
- **What are your differential diagnoses?**
  - Head lice may be confused with pubic lice (Phthirus pubis) or body lice (Pediculus humanus). They can be distinguished by the location where they are found: see the CKS topic on Pubic lice for more information.
  - Nits may be confused with seborrhoeic scales, hair muffs (secretions from the hair follicle that are wrapped round the hair shaft) and particles from hair products (such as hair spray). They can be distinguished by brushing the hair.
  - Itching is not always caused by an active head lice infestation:
  - It could also be caused by other itchy scalp conditions, such as eczema.
  - It may not develop for several weeks or months after the onset of infestation, or persist for days or weeks after successful eradication.
  - Itching is a common reaction to hearing that there are head lice within the school or community.
- **What clinical signs would enable you to make a diagnosis?**
  - Detection combing (the systematic combing of the hair with a fine-toothed head lice detection comb) is the most reliable way to confirm the presence of head lice, and it is much more reliable than visual inspection.
  - A live louse must be found in order to confirm active head lice infestation.
  - An itching scalp is not sufficient to diagnose active infestation.
  - The presence of louse eggs alone, whether hatched (nits) or unhatched, does not indicate active infestation.

Further reading and useful websites

While most of the consultation models explored in this chapter were traditionally for medical practitioners, the consultation model by Hastings and Redsall was developed specifically for nurses. It also includes a tool for self-assessing (or peer-assessing) competence in relation to your consultations. You may want to read this publication which includes some background to their consultation instrument; the tool itself that can be printed off and used in practice.

Hastings A. and Redsall S. (2006b) Using the Consultation Assessment and Improvement Instrument for Nurses (CAIIN) in Assessment (online). https://www.researchgate.net/publication/254757754_Using_the_Consultation_Assessment_and_Improvement_Instrument_for_Nurses_CAIIN_in_assessment

Activity 3.6 explored the concept of making a diagnosis in relation to head lice. You may wish to read further:

NICE Clinical Knowledge Summaries (CKS) (2018d) *Head Lice* (online). https://cks.nice.org.uk/head-lice

Chapter 4   Evidence-based practice and prescribing governance

RPS Competency Framework for All Prescribers (2021a)

This chapter will address the following professional competencies:

- **Competency 2: Identify evidence-based treatment options available for clinical decision-making**
- **Competency 4: Prescribe**
- **Competency 5: Provide information**
- **Competency 6: Monitor and review**
- **Competency 7: Prescribe safely**

NMC Future Nurse: Standards of Proficiency for Registered Nurses

This chapter will address the following platforms and proficiencies:

Platform 1: Being an accountable professional

At the point of registration, the registered nurse will be able to:

1.7   demonstrate an understanding of research methods, ethics and governance in order to critically analyse, safely use, share and apply research findings to promote and inform best nursing practice.

1.8   demonstrate the knowledge, skills and ability to think critically when applying evidence and drawing on experience to make evidence informed decisions in all situations.

Chapter aims

After reading this chapter, you will be able to:

- explain the key features and role of evidence-based practice within the context of prescribing practice;

(Continued)

(Continued)

- apply critical thinking and judicious use of evidence to inform person-centred prescribing decisions;
- identify pertinent guidelines and frameworks for prescribing while recognising limits to your scope of practice;
- identify contributors to governance such as care quality, improvement and reporting systems for prescribing.

Introduction

As in all areas of nursing practice, a professional, ethical and legal duty of care is owed to the people we may be making prescribing decisions for as underpinned by the Code (NMC, 2018a). This duty of care includes having the knowledge and skills to undertake a thorough assessment and a grasp of the various factors that inform shared decision-making. Undertaking an assessment involves having an awareness of physiology and pathophysiology, the condition(s) you are diagnosing, including the expected trajectory of its progression, and the recommended treatment options. All of these rely on clinical judgement, current knowledge, skills and expertise, along with an awareness of when you need to seek help or guidance from others.

Many conditions or prescribing decisions can be addressed through recognised care pathways, protocols, frameworks, clinical guidelines or prescribing formularies. This chapter uses clinical guidelines and pathways to exemplify the need to evaluate and appraise evidence and other influences on decision-making within your area of practice and this is no different when making prescribing decisions. It looks at the range of evidence sources to promote informed choice for the people you will be guiding towards clinical decisions. Being mindful that evidence is also needed to underpin assessment and diagnosis, the CASE acronym from the previous chapter is used to consider sources of evidence when selecting particular courses of action, such as prescribing, not prescribing, providing advice or de-prescribing. The need to use your judgement when applying evidence and guidelines is discussed, followed by further exploration of how to justify the information you provide for care decisions and the applicability of the evidence to the unique individual and their preferences.

These topics are considered in the context of achieving the best outcomes which must always put the person at the centre of decision-making. The topics also comprise the core features of clinical governance. Safe and effective care that meets standards and improves quality is at the centre of clinical governance. Prescribing governance is discussed in relation to standards, measurement, medication errors or **adverse events**, and systems for reporting or improvement.

Introduction to evidence-based practice

Sackett *et al.* (2000, p2) defined evidence-based practice as: *the conscientious, explicit and judicious use of current best evidence in making decisions about the care of individual patients.* This was added to by Strauss *et al.* (2019) who suggested it is a combination of best research evidence, a practitioner's own clinical expertise and knowledge, along with the person's unique values and circumstances. They also consider the person's values, expectations and priorities, as well as their physical presentation or clinical state when assessed (Strauss *et al.*, 2019). We often work with evidence that has been 'pre-appraised' to inform clinical guidelines, care protocols, the British National Formulary (BNF) (NICE, JFC) or Nurse Prescribers' Formulary (NPF) (NICE, AGNP). As illustrated in Figure 4.1, decisions are made in combination with our own and others' knowledge and experience; the perspective of the person in our care helps guide decision-making.

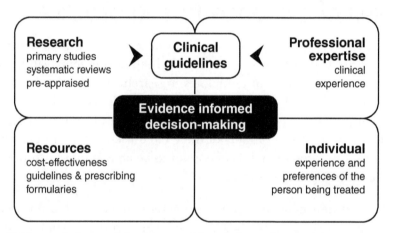

Figure 4.1 Evidence-informed decision-making (adapted from DiCenso *et al.*, 1998)

Evidence-informed decision-making

Activity 4.1 uses an example of childhood eczema to prompt you to think critically about what you currently know, how you know this and the sources of information you might use in practice.

Activity 4.1 Critical thinking

Cath has called about six-week-old Milly; she reports she has noticed dry skin for several weeks but it now seems to be getting worse and is itchy and sore-looking. While children may not be part of your area of care, think about how you might inform a diagnosis and recommend treatment. Consider the following.

(Continued)

(Continued)

- What are/were your first thoughts on this condition? How did you know this?
- What would you do if this was outside your scope of practice?
- What might influence your diagnosis and decision-making?
- How do you know what is best practice?

When answering Activity 4.1 you can apply the contributing factors of informed choice/ evidence-based practice to this scenario as shown in Figure 4.1.

Some suggested answers can be found at the end of this chapter within the answer to this activity.

Principles of evidence-based practice

In Activity 4.1, answers to the initial questions will vary greatly between practitioners. For example, those without any experience of childhood eczema will be highly reliant on information contained in guidelines, research literature or help from more experienced practitioners. In contrast, health visitors are likely to have encountered this regularly in practice, so have seen the usual pattern of presentation, treatments and their success or otherwise. In any of these circumstances, as a nurse advising the mother, or as a future prescriber, it is important to be able to explain your decisions or advice and the underpinning evidence.

Before applying evidence-based practice to decision-making about the specific products or treatment strategies (using the CASE acronym), the wider context and judicious use of evidence to also inform diagnosis should be considered. This section discusses some of the types of research evidence, with the aim of being able to explain decision-making. One way to think about it is to consider how you would present a rationale if you were informing a person about their treatment choices, or justifying a decision to your practice assessor, or even in a court of law. Being an autonomous practitioner entails having a grasp of the hierarchy of evidence and what it means for research to be considered valid, reliable and robust enough to underpin decisions. Some of the many sources of your knowledge and justification for practice decisions are illustrated in Figure 4.2.

Clinical guidelines and other pre-appraised evidence

While not all of the situations we encounter as nurses or future prescribers will be covered by clinical guidelines, a good range of these are available. The starting point for assessment, diagnosis and treatment options should normally be national and

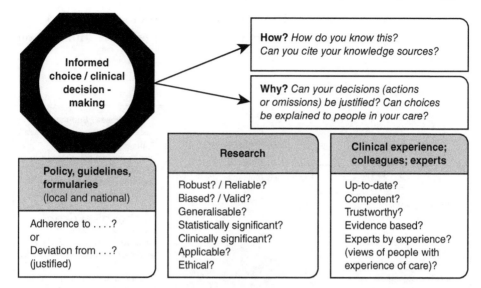

Figure 4.2 Informed choice and clinical decision-making

local guidelines, care protocols or prescribing formularies, including the BNF/NPF. Guidelines from the National Institute of Health and Care Excellence (NICE) or the Scottish Intercollegiate Guideline Network (SIGN) offer a reliable backing for the diagnosis and best practice to inform treatment options.

National guideline development typically involves a systematic review of original research and other literature and input from expert practitioners and service users, as well as an economic analysis (NICE, 2020a). Some guideline development has input from additional stakeholders, such as the royal colleges. Clinical guidelines and care protocols represent one type of 'pre-appraised' evidence and there are other forms that can be helpful for informing decision-making. While it is recognised we need to critically appraise primary research (such as drug trials), appraisal tools also exist for checking the strength of systematic reviews and it should not be assumed that these are all of the same high quality (DiCenso *et al.*, 2009; Strauss *et al.*, 2019).

Evidence sources

The 'traditional' hierarchy of evidence starts with the most subjective: 'mechanistic reasoning' (expert opinion), towards the more objective: case series, cohort studies, to randomised controlled trials and finally systematic reviews (Murad *et al.*, 2016). Some guidelines such as the Scottish Intercollegiate Guideline Network (SIGN, 2019) award the same grading to a single high-quality RCT as to a systematic review of RCTs. In 'pre-appraised' evidence pyramids, single primary studies are at the bottom with other forms of pre-appraised research higher up the scale (Alper and Haynes, 2016). Where possible, appraised research from reliable sources should be the first point of reference to underpin your decision-making alongside policies and protocols. Figure 4.3 outlines the main forms of primary and secondary (pre-appraised) evidence with an indication of their hierarchy.

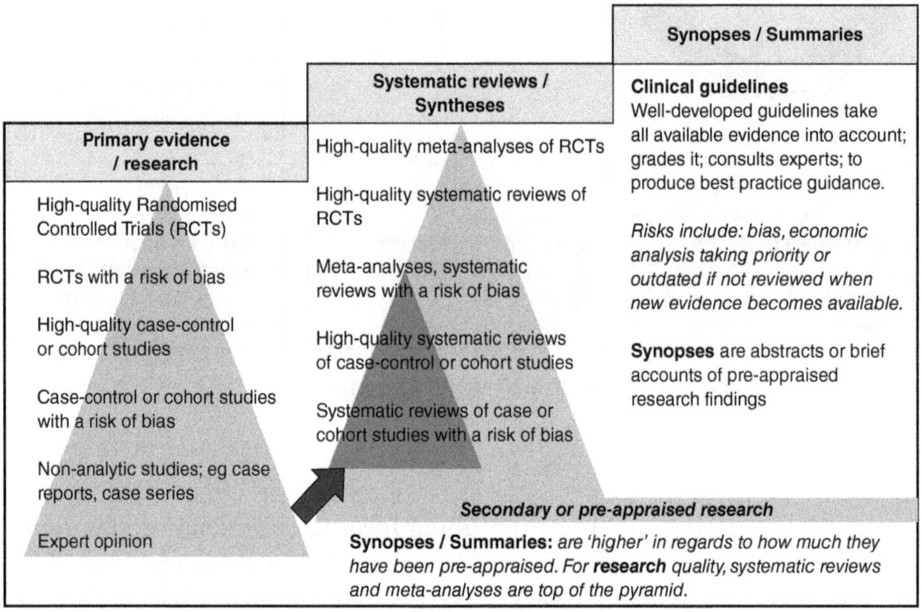

Synopses / Summaries

Systematic reviews / Syntheses

Clinical guidelines
Well-developed guidelines take all available evidence into account; grades it; consults experts; to produce best practice guidance.

Risks include: bias, economic analysis taking priority or outdated if not reviewed when new evidence becomes available.

Primary evidence / research

High-quality meta-analyses of RCTs

High-quality systematic reviews of RCTs

Synopses are abstracts or brief accounts of pre-appraised research findings

High-quality Randomised Controlled Trials (RCTs)

RCTs with a risk of bias

Meta-analyses, systematic reviews with a risk of bias

High-quality case-control or cohort studies

High-quality systematic reviews of case-control or cohort studies

Case-control or cohort studies with a risk of bias

Systematic reviews of case or cohort studies with a risk of bias

Non-analytic studies; eg case reports, case series

Secondary or pre-appraised research

Expert opinion

Synopses / Summaries: *are 'higher' in regards to how much they have been pre-appraised. For* **research** *quality, systematic reviews and meta-analyses are top of the pyramid.*

Figure 4.3   Hierarchy of primary and secondary evidence

(adapted from SIGN (2019) and Alper and Haynes (2016))

Best practice requires an awareness of the most up-to-date evidence. Seeking and applying primary research studies to inform choice and clinical decisions can be challenging due to the sheer volume, as well as the need to be certain the research is valid and robust. For pre-appraised research, the levels in Figure 4.3 correspond to how extensively the evidence has been integrated into clinical decision-making, with the least at the bottom and the highest integration at the top. Information sources are now outlined starting from the least appraised/integrated to the most.

Studies/synopsis of studies

Studies are primary research and investigations into specific clinical problems (e.g. a randomised trial of a new antimicrobial dressing). Synopses of studies (or reports of individual original research) can be found on websites that keep track of newly published research. Unlike evidence that is pre-appraised, research studies need to be assessed for how robust, reliable and free from bias the findings are. This critical appraisal is normally done using appraisal tools. The advantage of individual studies is that they are the first type of research to be published, so often represent the most up-to-date information. Clinical guidelines can take years to establish and although they are reviewed regularly, you may find some original research that answers a clinical question more correctly than the published guideline. This chapter doesn't extend to methods of appraising primary research, but it is important to remember that fulfilling your duty of care means being up to date with the most recent and robust evidence.

While primary studies need appraising, 'synopses' of studies have already been filtered and reviewed with the key content extracted. Ways of accessing extracts and keeping up to date include subscribing to medicines alerts or evidence updates for your area of practice. Some example websites are available at the end of this chapter as Further reading.

Systematic reviews/synopses of reviews

A systematic review is a detailed and thorough process that aims to identify, appraise and synthesise all the relevant primary evidence to answer a specific research question (Cochrane, 2020). Systematic reviews use protocols that explicitly outline the methods used for the review, so as to minimise bias, improve the reliability of the findings and make the process transparent. Reviews are used to inform decision-making by comprehensively finding evidence on a specific clinical question (e.g. dressings or topical agents for preventing pressure ulcers). Synopses of systematic reviews provide succinct summaries that are more easily applied to the clinical setting. These carefully edited, typically one- or two-page summaries provide an outline of the key findings on a specific clinical question. Systematic reviews/syntheses provide far more detail so are good sources of information for a topic that is unfamiliar. Examples are included in the Further reading at the end of the chapter.

Systematic guidelines/summaries

While systematic reviews focus on specific research questions, summaries address broader clinical topics, such as asthma or diabetes. Care pathways or systematic clinical guidelines also provide a summary of the best evidence but tend to be more focused (e.g. insulin for Type 1 diabetes). They offer evidence-based 'best practice' recommendations for clinical care. Some example links are found in Further reading. Activity 4.2 invites you to explore and compare evidence sources.

Activity 4.2   Finding evidence sources

Cath reports that the emollient isn't working for Milly's dry skin condition. It now seems to be worsening with even more itchiness and redness, and Milly has been increasingly irritable. She is seeking advice for something stronger than an emollient. Explore three

(Continued)

(Continued)

different sources of information and consider which would be most helpful if you needed to make a diagnosis of 'childhood eczema' and offer advice. It is acknowledged that in practice you would most likely need to refer or ask the help of your practice assessor, but the purpose of this activity is to compare evidence sources for their usefulness to practice. Some example sources are:

1. **The BNF, BNFc or NPF.**
2. **Summaries/systematic guidelines**.

   Clinical Knowledge Summaries: https://cks.nice.org.uk/eczema-atopic#!topicSummary

   SIGN (quick reference and full guidance): https://www.sign.ac.uk/our-guidelines/management-of-atopic-eczema-in-primary-care/

   NICE Pathway: https://pathways.nice.org.uk/pathways/eczema

3. **Summaries of studies/original studies**.

   NICE evidence search: https://www.evidence.nhs.uk/search?q=Childhood+Eczema

   Cochrane clinical answers: https://www.cochranelibrary.com/cca

There is no answer provided for Activity 4.2 but the links will provide you with a good overview of the different types of information available. This activity aims to prompt you to explore a topic which you may be unfamiliar with to help you consider how easy or otherwise the research information was to find and interpret. For any prescribing decision, it is imperative that you have a good grasp of the evidence underpinning assessment, diagnosis, and treatment options. Next, we look more closely at the considerations when promoting informed choice for treatment decisions.

Establishing a diagnosis and treatment aims

As discussed in Chapter 3 as part of the RAPID model, the end result of a thorough assessment is to establish a working diagnosis. As with the treatment options, the working diagnosis needs to be evidence-based, using established methods of assessment and diagnosis where possible. Even when the diagnosis has been affirmed, symptoms or conditions can change over time or it may transpire that the underlying cause or diagnosis was in error. Some conditions are challenging to formally diagnose, so monitoring response to treatment is key. Furthermore, even when a diagnosis is confirmed, there is a need to agree the treatment aims with the person in your care. For example, an assumption can be made that a person with a chronic leg wound has the aim of the wound being healed. However, if psycho-social factors take priority, they may unconsciously or otherwise have the aim of continuing with a wound so as to maintain regular contact with a healthcare professional. Conversely, wound healing may be an aim but comfort and mobility is prioritised due to an underlying condition. Activity 4.3 asks you to think critically about treatment aims.

Activity 4.3   Critical thinking: influences on treatment aims

Mrs Smith's daughter contacts you to assess her mother's leg wound as it appears she is in discomfort and reportedly scratching at her dressings. On arrival, it is clear that the wound has worsened, the surrounding skin is warm to touch and Mrs Smith is in discomfort. She says she doesn't want any more of those horrible tight bandages as they are making it worse. What might influence the treatment aims?

Some suggestions are found at the end of this chapter.

Activity 4.3 serves as a reminder that we sometimes need to consider immediate treatment aims, the perspective and priorities of those who are being cared for and the longer-term implications for treatment decisions. The next section looks at influences on treatment decisions as part of the CASE for your prescribing.

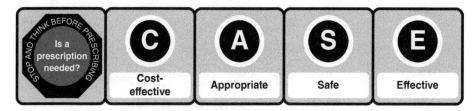

Figure 4.4   CASE

Now that we have looked at some of the evidence sources, we will reconsider practical treatment decisions in line with whether the product or treatment choice is **C**ost-effective, **A**ppropriate, **S**afe and **E**ffective.

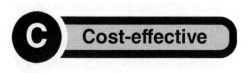

Cost-effective

The cost of prescriptions on the NHS is substantial, making it an important concern. Resources need to be distributed equitably with optimum use of the NHS budget, while fulfilling our duty of care. NICE and other guidelines undertake economic analyses and sometimes, after weighing the available evidence, the costs become a priority over other factors. Your selection of products or medicines is normally based on local formularies that have been derived from national guidelines. This provides a solid base from which you can select appropriate treatment options. However, disadvantages revolve around potential ethical dilemmas if you are aware of better evidence for a more costly product or treatment, or if the person being prescribed for expresses a clear preference. The ethical dilemmas of providing person-centred best practice, or being convinced the extra cost will save resources in the longer term need consideration. You can prescribe outside the local formulary or guidelines but will need to communicate this appropriately and be prepared to provide a strong rationale for this decision. Organisations should have a mechanism by which you can apply for an exemption, or recommend a treatment that is not currently on the formulary. Local formularies are normally based on national guidelines, but can take local variation into account. For example, a higher rate of bacterial resistance to the usual front-line treatment can prompt a different antibiotic on the local formulary.

Another strategy is to provide a rationale through research, cost analysis and/or clinical audit. An example of this is expensive alternative methods of compression therapy not available on most formularies. Some products are much more expensive than tradition four-layer bandages, but due to ease of application they are potentially cost-saving and can promote independence or self-care. While they may not be on local formularies, or only prescribed in special circumstances, examples exist where a community-wide cost–benefits analysis was used to demonstrate overall saving. Through audit and action, it is possible to get products added to your local formulary.

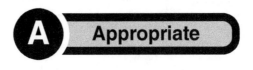

Appropriate

When considering if a treatment choice is suitable for the individual, factors such as pre-existing medical conditions, age, renal function, liver function, known allergies and potential drug interactions need to be taken into account. It is necessary to have an awareness of all the medications the person is taking, even if most of these are outside your scope of prescribing practice. Attentiveness to the risks of interactions or adverse drug effects is the responsibility of all prescribers (RPS, 2021a). An appropriate evidence base in most cases is the British National Formulary which is available as an app or online resource from NICE. Another source of detailed, up-to-date and approved information on all medicines available in the UK is the electronic Medicines Compendium (eMC). This includes summaries of product characteristics (SPCs or SmPCs) and patient information leaflets (PILs). The eMC resource also holds information in the form of risk minimisation materials (RMMs). Along with assuring there are no **contra-indications** or potential interactions, the eMC and BNF can also help you select the right product, dose, formulation and the duration of treatment as appropriate for the individual.

It must be noted that special caution is advised when prescribing in pregnant or breastfeeding women as certain drugs may be harmful to the foetus or are excreted in breastmilk, so unless you are a midwife, these are likely outside your scope of practice. The RCN (2021a) has issued guidance for nurse independent prescribers that suggests they do not prescribe for any pregnancy-related condition. While they suggest a useful distinction may be whether the 'condition' being treated by the prescriber is related to the pregnancy or not; even then they suggest a referral to the midwifery team, GP or consultant, as appropriate.

Age is another important consideration. The children's BNF (NICE, JFC) states medicines should only be prescribed for children when they are necessary, and it is always important to consider the risks. An awareness is needed of the differences of children's response to drugs, particularly neonates (NICE, JFC). Professionally, there is an expectation that nurses only prescribe within their scope of practice (NMC, 2018a, b; RPS, 2021a). This involves nurses being aware of the anatomical, physiological and developmental differences when prescribing for children, as this is considered a specialist or distinct area of practice.

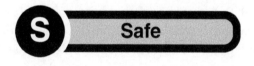

Safe

In addition to the person-specific cautions, most treatment options involve some risk of harm or adverse reaction so resources such as the BNF or eMC should be considered. Responsibilities include keeping in touch with new evidence, alerts or warnings, so you should subscribe to regular updates. These updates may highlight new reported reactions with the information reliant on practitioners reporting these. Suspected or confirmed adverse drug reactions are normally escalated with a course of action determined – for example, stop the drug, reduce the dose or treat the side effect. NICE CKS (2018c) suggests it is important to assess the nature and severity of the reaction in order to determine whether urgent action is required or whether the person can be managed safely in primary care. It provides specific examples, such as cough due to an angiotensin-converting enzyme inhibitor, as being relatively minor and commonly occurring, as opposed to a rare medical emergency like anaphylaxis.

Adverse drug effects should be reported through the Yellow Card system and noted on the person's medical record as appropriate. This helps inform the evidence for medicinal products and can lead to medications being withdrawn. NICE CKS (2018c) states that all products indicated in the BNF with a black triangle need to be reported, as these are new drugs and vaccines that are being intensively monitored by the MHRA to confirm their risk/benefit profile. Black triangle drugs represent the latter stages of the research process whereby they have been tested and licensed for use, but need to pass this final stage to be deemed to be broadly safe in practice.

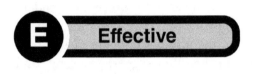

Effective

The NPC (1999a) advice regarding prescribing effectively suggests that nurses who are V100 prescribers should be familiar with the full range of items in the Nurse Prescribers' Formulary (NPF) to help ensure that the most appropriate prescription item is selected. While this may be appropriate for a limited formulary it is not realistic for prescribers with access to the full formulary, and there is still a need to be able to highlight the clinical effectiveness of one product over another. The NPC (1999a) recognised that even those prescribing from the NPF should critically appraise the available evidence to assess the product's effectiveness. The NPF is not updated frequently so should be used in tandem with the most recent BNF along with guidance and research that attempts to quantify their effectiveness. The aim is to avoid subjectivity so that decisions can be seen as independently verifiable.

We previously discussed the benefits of guidelines and other forms of pre-appraised evidence. However, the Oxford Centre for Evidence-Based Medicine (OCEBM) suggests that while these evidence sources may be more comprehensive, they risk reliance on expert authority. The centre encourages medical practitioners to appraise original research themselves (Howick *et al.*, 2011) and suggests also considering the following questions before concluding the treatment that should be used.

- Is there good reason to believe that the person you are prescribing for is sufficiently similar to the people in the studies examined?
- Does the treatment have a clinically relevant benefit that outweighs the harms?
- Is another treatment better?
- Are the patient's values and circumstances compatible with the treatment?

(Howick *et al.*, 2011)

Activity 4.4 asks you to consider what sources of information you will likely be using when prescribing or providing advice in your area of practice.

> ## Activity 4.4   Reflection: evidence-based prescribing
>
> Thinking about your area of future prescribing practice, what are some of the sources of information you would use to guide:
>
> * evidence-based prescribing?
> * information to help the person with their treatment decisions?
> * cautions, side effects and safety-netting advice?
>
> *There is no answer provided as this is specific to your area of practice.*

Clinical governance and prescribing practice

We have discussed the pertinence of evidence-based sources of information for diagnosis and decision-making, and touched on governance mechanisms such as standardised formularies and adverse drug reaction reporting. These processes are necessary both for patient safety in the wider sense and to help you learn from and improve your personal prescribing practice. 'Clinical governance' is a broad term that relates to any activities that help to enhance the quality of care provided. Scally and Donaldson (1998) define it as a basis for organisations to uphold high standards by *creating an environment in which excellence in clinical care will flourish.* Front-line staff have a responsibility to contribute to processes that help assure high-quality care. The RPS (2019) suggests that clinical governance involves recognising and upholding good practice, learning from mistakes and improving quality.

In relation to medicines management and prescribing, this includes activities such as observing policies, safe storage, transport and administration of medicines, along with documentation, reporting and auditing errors, reviewing practice and participating in continuing professional development. Improvement mechanisms for practitioners and organisations include adverse drug reaction reporting (using the Yellow Card system); incident, error and near miss reporting; analysing prescribing data (including prescription costs); clinical audit; developing policies; procedures and formularies; and issuing, communicating or acting upon alerts and warnings.

Activity 4.5 uses an example of an adverse reaction in relation to the treatment of childhood eczema to prompt you to think critically about some of the reporting and governance mechanisms in prescribing practice.

Activity 4.5 Critical thinking: adverse reaction reporting

Cath has called again about her baby Milly and reports that she has tried the prescribed emollient for three days. She is quite worried as Milly's skin condition is looking worse and seems quite red, itchy, sore and inflamed. Your practice assessor has seen these symptoms previously and suspects it may be a sensitivity reaction to the emollient.

- What would be the first course of action or advice?
- What reporting or referral might need to be made?
- How might you and the team learn from this?

Some suggested answers to Activity 4.5 can be found at the end of the chapter.

Applying clinical governance to your prescribing practice

An outline of some of the mechanisms contributing to improving quality and assuring standards has been provided. This section highlights a selection of these in more detail and with reference to some of the recognised resources or tools to help implement clinical governance. The topics include: policy, protocols and formularies; clinical audit; medication errors; adverse drug reactions; and medicines optimisation. The example of antimicrobial stewardship is used to illustrate some of these.

Policies, care protocols, formularies

To improve the quality of care, various guidelines have been developed that often translate locally into policies and care protocols that nurses need to follow when prescribing, supplying or administering medications. These aim to raise the standard of care, reduce risk of adverse events and provide a baseline against which care can be measured. Examples include: patient group directives, protocols for sepsis, wound care or local prescribing formularies. As a prescriber, these are important not only for selecting the most appropriate product, but also in providing advice or promoting informed choice, and considering whether systems are in place to assure the treatment is safely delivered or administered. Cost savings are often a concern when formularies or protocols are being developed, so competing priorities can impact on decisions as to whether to adhere to or deviate from these.

Activity 4.6 involves accessing the prescribing policy within your practice setting and using an example of childhood eczema, or another example of your choice, to prompt you to think critically about some of the competing demands when expected to adhere to guidelines, protocols or formularies.

Activity 4.6   Critical thinking

Cath has returned to clinic with Milly and reports there has been no improvement since she was prescribed a mild steroidal cream the day before. She is convinced Milly's skin condition is infected since not only is it still red, sore and inflamed, but there is some weeping too. Your practice assessor suspects it may be just be a matter of giving time for the steroidal cream to take effect, but Cath is adamant she wants antibiotics to be prescribed.

- What would be the first course of action or advice?
- What are some of the key policies or protocols that would guide this decision?
- What are some of the ethical aspects of this decision?

Some suggested answers to Activity 4.6 can be found at the end of the chapter.

Clinical audit

Audits check whether care standards are being implemented as they start with a standard statement and measure against this. For example, a standard in the hospital setting may be that 100 per cent of medications are administered within two hours of the stated time. There are specific audit tools that aid data collection to measure this. In the community setting, there can also be documentation audits. The key features of an audit identify the standard(s) against which practice is measured, collect the data or information and, where needed, recommend actions to improve upon current practice. Re-auditing is then a way to measure if these improvements have occurred. While organisations often design audits, smaller team units such as a community nursing team can benefit from designing their own audits for the same purpose of improving practice.

Activity 4.7 uses an example of an observation in practice that results in a team undertaking an audit for the purposes of improving care outcomes.

Activity 4.7   Critical thinking: audit

You are working in a busy community nursing team with many people being seen because of their long-term wounds. There is a new team leader and she has noticed there seem to be more people with diabetic foot ulcers or amputations than she has previously seen. She is not certain why this is, so has worked with the team to undertake an audit.

- Where would she look for a standard around diabetic foot care?
- What type of questions might an audit ask?
- What would the aim be?

Some suggested answers to Activity 4.7 can be found at the end of the chapter.

Medication errors: risk management and incident reporting

A medication error is defined by the European Medicines Agency (2014) as *an unintended failure in the drug treatment process that leads to, or has the potential to lead to, harm.* This includes any error in the process of prescribing, preparing, dispensing, administering, monitoring or providing advice on medicines (CQC, 2021). These patient safety incidents can generally be divided into two categories; errors of commission or errors of omission. The former includes for example, wrong medicine or wrong dose (CQC, 2021). Although most medication errors occur at the administration stage, it is important to be vigilant as a prescriber in ensuring prescriptions are legible, accurate and given with clear instructions (RPS, 2021a).

NHS Improvement (2018a) suggests that *recording incidents protects patients from harm and saves lives.* Reporting aims to identify the nature of errors to help improve systems and reduce the risk of errors occurring. In England, the National Reporting and Learning System (NRLS) (NHS Improvement, 2018a) records safety incidents and defines these as *any unintended or unexpected incident, which could have or did lead to harm.* The Patient Safety Incident Management System (PSIMS) is a replacement for the NRLS. The aim of the PSIMS is to make reporting more efficient with automated uploads from local systems; allow centralised online reporting for non-hospital care settings; and collect more useful data that will be easier to access by local teams. For more information about incident reporting systems please see Further reading.

Under-reporting of medication errors is a notable problem, with only 0.1 per cent of estimated total medication errors being reported. Using projected figures, Elliot *et al.* (2018) calculated 237 million medication errors per year, with 66 million of these potentially clinically significant. While this study was based on the English NHS, medication error is viewed as a global problem, with the World Health Organization (WHO) aiming to activate improvements in patient safety worldwide. WHO (2017) identify that medication errors occur *when weak medication systems and/or human factors such as fatigue, poor environmental conditions or staff shortages affect prescribing, transcribing, dispensing, administration and monitoring practices, which can then result in severe harm, disability and even death.* Their launch of *'Medication Without Harm'* (WHO, 2017) aims to reduce the global burden of severe and avoidable medication-related harm, with three early priorities for action identified: high-risk situations, polypharmacy and transitions of care. As a practitioner involved with medicines and as a prescriber, you will need to be alert to the risks associated with these, as well as others you observe in practice. Activity 4.8 asks you to consider priorities for action to help address medication error.

Activity 4.8 Critical thinking: priority areas for medication errors

In response to the global challenge of medication errors, a working group in England was set up to identify priority areas for action. Think about some of the situations you may have witnessed in practice where there was an error, or a near miss? What would you see as priorities for action?

An outline answer giving the priorities identified is found at the end of the chapter.

Activity 4.8 looked at some priorities for action around medication error. Root cause analyses or serious case reviews are needed in certain circumstances and you should refer to your local guidelines for these. On a larger scale, there is a serious incident reporting process, which may need to be taken by the organisation in the event of significant harm or death occurring. Like the previously mentioned reporting systems, the purpose of these mechanisms is to identify and address issues that may be leading to errors or other causes of harm. Another source of potential harm is adverse drug reactions (ADRs). WHO (2002) define an **ADR** as *a response to a medicine which is noxious and unintended, and which occurs at doses normally used in man.* Reporting is an important part of clinical governance that leads to a body of information that can help reduce the risk of harm caused by medicinal products. When new drugs are involved, as denoted by a black triangle in the BNF, this can also be seen as research governance. Further advice around reporting adverse drug reactions can be found in the NICE Clinical Knowledge Summaries (NICE, 2018c).

The Medicines and Healthcare Products Regulatory Agency (MHRA) serves a clear governance function as they are responsible for the regulation of medicines, medical devices and blood components for transfusion in the UK. The agency has a public health protection and improvement role as well as promoting innovation through scientific research and development. The MHRA's role in medicines includes ensuring they meet applicable standards of safety, quality and efficacy, ensuring that the supply chain is safe and secure and helping to educate the public and healthcare professionals about the risks and benefits, leading to safer and more effective use. Practitioners should sign up for the regular MHRA safety alerts. There are other resources, governance and safety information on the MHRA website, including, for example, drug and safety alerts or updates, the Yellow Card reporting system, patient information leaflets and summaries of medicinal products, drug analysis prints and public assessment reports.

Chapter summary

This chapter explored evidence-based practice for treatment decisions, prescribing and advice giving. Clinical decision-making derives from a range of information, including,

(Continued)

(Continued)

among others, research literature, policy guidelines, expert opinion and the person's treatment aims and preferences. While evidence-based approaches should underpin decision-making, they are also important in the context of informed choice and achieving concordance. Clinical guidelines and local care protocols are examples of governance mechanisms, and normally comprise the best available evidence. The prescriber's role in contributing to and participating in clinical governance mechanisms to improve practice was outlined in this chapter. Taking ownership for recognising potentially risky situations; reporting incidents, errors and adverse reactions; identifying areas for improvement and acting upon these are all part of your clinical governance role.

Activities: suggested answers and discussion points

Answer to Activity 4.1 Critical thinking

Considering the scenario in Activity 4.1 we can apply evidence-based practice (EBP) to this scenario by considering each of the contributing factors shown in Figure 4.1.

- Your first thoughts: This relates to your current knowledge and experience. It may be that you have never encountered children before, but have previously seen and diagnosed adult eczema so can apply similar principles.
- Scope of practice: The expectation in any situation where you recognise limits to your scope of practice is to seek guidance and support from others. It may simply be that your job contract doesn't cover the care of children, or that you recognise the situation as requiring additional knowledge and skills.
- Influences on your diagnosis and decision-making/best practice: All four of the areas (1. Professional knowledge and experience; 2. Research; 3. The person's perspective; 4. Resources) will be an influence and, similarly, will combine to help you gather what is best practice in this situation. These are outlined in further detail.

1. **Professional knowledge/experience**: Your own previous experience or practice expertise may guide you in selecting an appropriate product. The scenario might be something you have encountered regularly in practice, or it could be as simple as knowing that a recommended product is not currently available due to a stock issue. Experience can be useful in the absence of guidelines, but you should still be able to articulate a rationale. Custom and practice does not always match current best evidence. For example, standard practice could be to prescribe only emollients for eczema, but a mild topical corticosteroid may also be needed (NICE CKS, 2021c).

2. **Research/evidence base**: Aside from the BNF/NPF, the first place to look is local policy, or recommended products from an approved formulary. As there is scant research evidence separating one emollient from another, the selection of specific products may be for other reasons such as cost. While the BNF/NPF are also evidence-based sources of information they don't provide enough detail to inform diagnosis or decision-making. For a common condition like eczema, it is possible to use gold standard resources including NICE or SIGN guidelines. For this condition (but not all) you can also start with the NICE Clinical Knowledge Summaries as these quickly identify the standard treatment regimens as well as making reference to the most up-to-date evidence to support these. See https://cks.nice.org.uk/

   Research and evidence are an important aid to informed choice. When providing advice, whether for non-pharmacological treatments (such as advising re. soap or laundry detergents), over the counter preparations, or prescription-only medicines, it is important to ensure that resources used are reputable and up to date. For example, you could guide the mum towards NHS Choices (https://www.nhs.uk/conditions/atopic-eczema/).

3. **Previous experience/preferences of the person being treated**: The mother may have used something previously for herself or other children and have a preconceived idea of what she would like to use in this instance. The people we prescribe for sometimes find new treatments before they are made widely available. There may also be preferences to take into account such as avoiding animal products, excipients or preservatives. There may be conflict between identified best practice and what is requested. For example, in one community, olive oil was being used by parents to treat infant eczema. The prescribing practitioners needed to be supportive and tactful, but also firm because of the duty of care owed to the infant.

4. **Resources**: This can be a major influence on decision-making, yet practitioners can feel they have little control over this. Resources include staff, equipment, treatments, products and medicines. If a resource is limited or not available, then alternative options must be considered. The most obvious examples of this are particular medications that haven't gained NICE approval, are limited by the local formulary ('post code lottery') or are out of stock. This also extends to treatments where staff shortages prevent the service from being available – for example, extended waiting lists for specialist mental health treatments such as CBT, creating a need for medication. The lack of resources may require different advice or treatments to be given.

Answer to Activity 4.3 Critical thinking: influences on treatment aims

Treatment priorities for Mrs Smith in this scenario should start with the 'Red, Amber, Green' outlined in Chapter 3, as it is advisable to first rule out any red flags or serious causes for concern. Wound infection can lead to sepsis, which can account for a deterioration in mental health (delirium states). The next consideration would be wound care assessment, the assessment tools you would use and establishing what is acceptable and preferable to Mrs Smith. In the short term, a mild infection or colonisation may be causing discomfort so she may need appropriate analgesia and a wound swab. Assessing quality of life helps shift the focus from being solely on physical assessment to addressing the wider impact (Green *et al.*, 2018a). Identifying priorities for Mrs Smith should be through a combination of what you understand of best practice for each phase of her condition in tandem with her preferences and treatment aims. In the short term, this may be promoting comfort, while longer term it may be to promote healing.

Answer to Activity 4.5 Critical thinking: adverse reaction reporting

*   **What would be the first course of action or advice?**
    Milly would require a visit or clinic appointment, either with the GP or your practice assessor, depending on her experience and scope of practice. The emollient should be stopped and there may now be a clinical need for a mild steroidal cream. As steroid cream is a POM, not in the NPF, this may require an appointment with the GP or a V300 prescriber rather than a V100/V150 prescriber.

*   **What reporting or referral might need to be made?**
    The adverse reaction should be recorded in Milly's care record and, depending on the circumstances, may need to be reported via the Yellow Card system. Some of the influences on this include the following.

    o   Is there any evidence or precedence for this issue? Is this a noted side effect? Some emollients are recognised as having excipients that can cause sensitivity reactions.
    o   Was the emollient a 'black triangle' medication (meaning that all reactions should be reported)?
    o   Was the reaction severe?
    o   Were there any alerts for this particular product?

*   **How might you and the team learn from this?**
    It is suggested that this is something the practice assessor has encountered before. It could be useful to undertake a brief scoping exercise to see how often this has occurred in the recent past. This could be set up more stringently as an audit to attempt to determine the prescribing trends of those on the team and if a specific emollient has caused more reactions than others. The use of practice level prescribing data (PACT) data can help with this.

Answer to Activity 4.6 Critical thinking

What would be the first course of action or advice?

Both SIGN (2011) and CKS (NICE CKS, 2021c) guidelines on atopic eczema highlight that one of the complications can be bacterial, herpetic or fungal infection. SIGN (2011, p15) has noted that *the skin lesions of around 90% of patients with atopic eczema are colonised with staphylococcus aureus compared to less than 5% of individuals with healthy skin*. Thus, the first action would be to rule out an infection. If this is not possible, the actions would depend on how unwell Milly is, as the guidelines (NICE, 2017b) suggest if there are signs of secondary infection – such as the patches weeping, being crusted, or having pustules, and there is fever or malaise – antibiotic treatment should be prescribed. NICE CKS (2021c) outlines the advice that should be offered, including the symptoms of infection and the potential medical emergency of 'eczema herpeticum' that requires immediate admission to hospital if suspected.

If infection can be ruled out, the question would then be around providing sensitive advice for self-care of the condition, aiming to reduce anxiety while explaining why antibiotics are not needed. For the purposes of the remaining answers, it is assumed that infection has been ruled out, with a focus on antimicrobial stewardship.

What are some of the key policies or protocols that would guide this decision?

The SIGN (2011) and Clinical Knowledge Summaries (NICE CKS) guidance covers swabbing, treatment, infection recurrence and the use of topical antibacterial preparations. There may also be local guidelines you can refer to, ideally linked to new research and/or expert opinion as guidelines are slow to be updated. CKS (NICE CKS 2021c) and SIGN (2011) suggest the use of topical antibiotics to treat localised areas of infection for up to two weeks (although research evidence is lacking), but are clear that oral antibiotics are not recommended in the treatment of non-infected eczema. Policies and protocols linked to antimicrobial stewardship are pertinent. NICE (2016a) has an 'antimicrobial stewardship' quality standard that aims to measure against quality statements to improve the structure, process and outcomes of care.

What are some of the ethical aspects of this decision?

It is recognised that eczema can cause stress and anxiety for people affected, and in this case, for the carer (NICE CKS, 2021c). In the absence of a clear infection, and in adherence to guidelines, the prescriber may need to oppose the wishes of the person in their care. We can look at this in line with some of the ethical principles outlined in Chapter 2.

Beneficence: standards and best practice protocols/guidance suggest it is most effective to treat non-infected eczema with emollients and steroidal creams (as needed). It is also of benefit to avoid overuse of antibiotics to reduce the likelihood of resistance if antibiotics were needed for Milly in the future.

Non-maleficence: not prescribing antibiotics reduces the risk of harm caused by side effects, allergic reactions or bacterial resistance. Conversely, if local colonisation progressed to a systemic infection, there is a risk of sepsis.

Justice: using guidelines supports fair, equal and standardised treatment or advice across the health service.

Autonomy: there is more of a conflict with promoting autonomy as the expressed wish of the parent is that antibiotics are prescribed. However, knowledge can be seen to increase autonomy, or at least informed choice. It may be that even after a clear, evidence-based rationale is provided, she still insists on antibiotics being prescribed. Depending on the circumstance, some prescribers, particularly doctors, may decide to support the parent's wishes, whether or not this can be clinically justified.

Utilitarianism vs deontology: this larger dilemma is one that policies (standards/formularies) attempt to address by weighing up the greatest good for the most people, and our duty to the individual. Policies around antimicrobial stewardship address both as it is neither good for an individual or the wider public for resistance to occur. However, there may be specific circumstances whereby not prescribing affects your duty to that individual. For example, if the eczema wasn't clinically infected at this time, but they were at risk of worsening and had difficulties accessing services.

Answer to Activity 4.7 Critical thinking: audit

Where would she look for a standard around wound assessment and care?

As this started with an observation, the first aim would be to provide evidence that this is a verifiable concern. This would be followed by attempting to ascertain the reason(s) and ideally be able to show improvement after making changes to practice. There is a national audit (for England and Wales) that covers the basic structure of care services, the management of those presenting with active diabetic foot disease, and their outcomes. The National Diabetes Foot Care Audit (NDFA) (NHS Digital, 2019b) seeks to address three key questions:

- **Structures**: Are the nationally recommended care structures in place for the management of diabetic foot disease?
- **Processes**: Does the treatment of active diabetic foot disease comply with nationally recommended guidance?
- **Outcomes**: Are the outcomes of diabetic foot disease optimised?

Standards relating to diabetic foot care are contained within guidelines on diabetes care (SIGN, 2017), or separate guidelines (Allam *et al.*, 2018; NICE, 2019a). The national audit (NHS Digital, 2019b) estimates approximately 20 per cent (or over 60,000 people in England) will have a diabetic foot ulcer, but acknowledges the number of new ulcers is not precisely known. Some statistics are available on healing times (35 per cent at 12 months, Guest *et al.*, 2018) and amputation rates (17 per cent at 12 months, Guest *et al.*, 2018). This suggests a simple measure against which to assess whether the observation is supported by data.

What type of questions might an audit ask? Once it was established the healing or amputation rates are worse than a comparable population, the audit questions would centre on best practice standard statements. Some examples include:

- all patients with diabetes should be screened to assess their risk of developing a foot ulcer (SIGN, 2017);
- prompt referral to a specialist multi-disciplinary foot team (MDFT) within one working day to reduce the risk of amputation and cost of treatment (NICE, 2015a);
- foot care education is recommended as part of a multi-disciplinary approach in all patients with diabetes (SIGN, 2017).

What would the aim be?

As with any audit, the underlying purpose would be to improve care quality and outcomes. The assessing and measurement of current practice can help identify areas for development, such as staff training, education, or access to resources or services. Re-audit should be undertaken to show if improvements had occurred.

Answer to Activity 4.8 Critical thinking: priority areas for medication errors

The Department of Health and Social Care (2018a) outlined these recommendations to help meet the global challenge of reducing medication errors, identifying that early priorities should include:

- improved **shared decision-making**;
- improve medication information for patients and families;
- encouraging and supporting patients and families to raise any concerns about their medication;

- improved shared care between health and care professionals; with increased knowledge and support;
- professional regulators must ensure **adequate training** in safe and effective medicines use is embedded in **undergraduate training**, and ensure continuing professional development adequately reflects safe and effective medicines use;
- professional regulators and professional leadership bodies should also encourage **reporting and learning from medication errors**;
- work with industry and MHRA to produce more patient-friendly **packaging and labelling**.

Further reading and useful websites

As discussed in this chapter, a range of useful resources are available. For evidence-based practice, these are grouped as: 1. EBP and research alerts; 2. Synopses, reviews and summaries and 3. Critical appraisal tools.

1. Evidence-based practice resources and research alerts

   - BMJ alerts. https://www.bmj.com/alerts
   - Evidence alerts. https://www.evidencealerts.com
   - NICE evidence. https://www.evidence.nhs.uk

2. Synopses, systematic reviews and summaries of best evidence

   - Centre for reviews and dissemination. https://www.york.ac.uk/crd/
   - Cochrane Library. https://www.cochranelibrary.com
   - Cochrane clinical answers. https://www.cochranelibrary.com/cca/about
   - British Medical Journal best practice. https://bestpractice.bmj.com/info/
   - NICE Clinical Knowledge Summaries. https://cks.nice.org.uk/
   - NICE guidelines. https://www.nice.org.uk
   - Scottish Intercollegiate Guidelines Network (SIGN). http://www.sign.ac.uk

3. Critical appraisal tools and information about research evidence.

   For information about critical appraisal, levels of evidence, evidence-based medicine tools and resources, the following are useful references:

   - Bandolier: Provides a glossary of research terms. http://www.bandolier.org.uk/glossary.html
   - CASP. (critical appraisal tools): https://casp-uk.net/casp-tools-checklists/
   - Centre for Evidence-based Medicine (CEBM) Critical Appraisal tools. https://www.cebm.net/2014/06/critical-appraisal/
   - PubMed also offer some short online tutorials and guides to basic evidence searches. https://learn.nlm.nih.gov/rest/training-packets/T0042010P.html

Clinical governance resources

This chapter also discussed clinical governance. Recommended reading includes information about medicines optimisation, prescribing data and safety alerts.

- NHS Business Services Authority (NHSBSA). https://www.nhsbsa.nhs.uk/prescription-data

  Records are kept on prescribing in England within all settings. This can be useful for noting the risks, types of medicines most commonly dispensed, and for improving prescribing practice. Data also covers some specific categories of prescribing.

- Prescribing data. https://openprescribing.net

  Prescribing across the NHS in England in a more accessible format. This can help. You compare your own prescribing with the national picture.

- MHRA. https://www.gov.uk/government/organisations/medicines-and-healthcare-products-regulatory-agency

  The Medicines and Healthcare Products Regulatory Agency (MHRA) regulates medicines, medical devices and blood components for transfusion in the UK. MHRA is an agency, sponsored by the Department of Health and Social Care. This is where you report adverse drug events (Yellow Card system), sign up for Drug and Device Safety Alerts and can find Drug Safety Updates.

- Yellow Card Centre (reporting and training, Scotland).

  https://www.yccscotland.scot.nhs.uk

- Health Improvement Scotland.

  https://ihub.scot/
  https://www.healthcareimprovementscotland.org/our_work/governance_and_assurance.aspx

Incident reporting and medicines safety

England

The National Patient Safety Improvement Programmes

https://www.england.nhs.uk/patient-safety/patient-safety-improvement-programmes/

NHS England: national patient safety alerts:

https://www.england.nhs.uk/patient-safety/national-patient-safety-alerting-committee/

NHS England: Patient Safety Incident Management System:

https://www.england.nhs.uk/patient-safety/patient-safety-incident-management-system/

Scotland

https://www.nss.nhs.scot/browse/health-facilities/incidents-and-alerts

Northern Ireland

Transforming Medication Safety in Northern Ireland

https://www.health-ni.gov.uk/publications/transforming-medication-safety-northern-ireland

Safety and Quality Standards

https://www.health-ni.gov.uk/topics/safety-and-quality-standards

Wales

Patient safety

https://du.nhs.wales/patient-safety-wales/

Chapter 5 Pharmacology and prescribing

Jill Gould, Alan Bloomer and Barry Strickland-Hodge

RPS Competency Framework for All Prescribers (2021a)

This chapter will address the following professional competencies:

- **Competency 2: Identify evidence-based treatment options available for clinical decision-making**
- **Competency 4: Prescribe**
- **Competency 5: Provide information**

NMC Future Nurse: Standards of Proficiency for Registered Nurses

This chapter will address the following platforms and proficiencies:

Platform 4: Providing and evaluating care

At the point of registration, the registered nurse will be able to:

4.15 demonstrate knowledge of pharmacology and the ability to recognise the effects of medicines, allergies, drug sensitivities, side effects, contra-indications, incompatibilities, adverse reactions, prescribing errors and the impact of polypharmacy and over the counter medication usage.

4.17 apply knowledge of pharmacology to the care of people, demonstrating the ability to progress to a prescribing qualification following registration.

Chapter aims

After reading this chapter, you will be able to:

- outline general principles of how drugs work and their importance in prescribing practice;

- explain how absorption, distribution, metabolism and excretion affect the action of a drug;
- describe how interactions, side effects and adverse drug reactions may occur and how to avoid or minimise risk.

Introduction

Scenario: Mr Jan

While in hospital, 85-year-old Mr Jan was given nystatin to treat the oral candidiasis he developed after a stroke. When you and your practice assessor visit him at home, he said it was no better, so miconazole oral gel was prescribed. When you revisit Mr Jan a few days later, he has some bruises visible on his arms. It transpires he was started on warfarin in hospital, but this was not updated on his medication list. You check the British National Formulary (BNF, JFC) and find that miconazole can greatly increase the anticoagulant effect of warfarin, so he is advised to stop taking the miconazole. However, on a subsequent visit, his bruising is worse and you discover his carers have continued to administer the oral gel.

Nurses are accountable for their clinical decisions and for the delegation of care to be provided by others. Responsibility as a prescriber includes being aware of others' prescribing and extends to the administration of medicines or application of products by others. To fulfil this duty of care, prescribers require sound clinical knowledge to inform evidence-based treatment options (NMC, 2018a). Medicines are the main treatment intervention used within healthcare and therefore safe decision-making also relies on a good grasp of pharmacology. A good foundation in pharmacological principles enhances safety, particularly with respect to drugs that act systemically. It is unrealistic to expect to know everything about all medicines, so it is recommended that you build a personal formulary as you gain a rounded understanding of the drugs you may be prescribing, administering or advising on. It is also important to know where to find reliable sources of information, starting with the British National Formulary (NICE, JFC), as well as other resources to expand your knowledge of pharmacology. Further resources can be found at the end of this chapter.

Pharmacology is a science that looks at the composition, effects and uses of drugs. It is normally split into how the body processes a drug (**pharmacokinetics**) and what effect the drug has on the body (**pharmacodynamics**) (Ritter and Rang, 2019). A good awareness of pharmacology and therapeutics will help with decisions regarding the choice of drug or product, route of administration, dose, cautions, advice, or follow-up care. It will also help you understand why drug doses, frequency of administration, contra-indications, side effects and interactions change depending on the drug and the individual. This chapter uses a scenario and clinical examples throughout to discuss core principles of basic pharmacology. It starts by asking you to think about what an 'ideal' medicine would look like. This is followed by an overview of routes of administration and the four pharmacokinetic processes of **ADME** (**absorption**, **distribution**, **metabolism** and **excretion**). A discussion of pharmacodynamics or how drugs act on the body follows. The majority of people we prescribe for require more than one medicinal product, so the topics of drug interactions and adverse drug reactions conclude the chapter.

Scenario: Mr Madiba Obi

You have been working with your practice assessor who is a practice nurse and independent (V300) prescriber. One of the people who attends her clinics regularly is Mr Madiba Obi, a 78-year-old with multiple long-term conditions. He prefers to be called by his first name, Madiba. He experiences knee pain because of arthritis, for which he is regularly using ibuprofen.

Activity 5.1 asks you to think about the scenario in relation to these questions. As we go through the chapter, we will revisit Madiba's scenario and consider it in more detail. We recommend the BNF (https://bnf.nice.org.uk) as the first point of reference.

Activity 5.1   Critical thinking

- What formulations of ibuprofen are available?
- How do you know which formulation Madiba should use and how much?
- What advice would Madiba need to be given to take ibuprofen safely?
- What side effects or adverse effects might he experience?
- Are there any concerns regarding Madiba taking ibuprofen and how may these be reduced?
- Is this a prescribed medicine? Is there a difference in prescribing ibuprofen between a community (V100/V150) and full formulary/non-medical (V300) prescriber?
- If not prescribed, how else might Madiba have obtained ibuprofen?

A short example answer is provided at the end of the chapter.

Medicines, risk and pharmacology

Various medicinal preparations have been used across the ages with modern science being able to better identify and extract active ingredients or synthesise new products.

Research helps to ascertain the action(s) and the unwanted effects of medicines. Despite insights provided by experience and research, basics such as the mechanisms of action remain unknown for some preparations while people react differently to medicines, so the emphasis is on continually observing and reporting, which we call pharmacovigilance. For example, despite paracetamol being one of the world's most commonly used drugs, first produced in 1878, its mechanism of action is not yet fully understood and is thought to involve a number of pathways (Sharma and Mehta, 2014; eMC, 2020).

One way to approach the topic of pharmacology is to think about the key features of a 'perfect' drug. Important attributes include being safe, selective to where it works on the body, effective, predictable in how it works, reversible in its action, easy to administer, free from interactions and cost effective. Looking at how medicines fall short of these attributes helps to explain why **pharmacovigilance** (the monitoring, understanding and prevention of adverse effects) is as important as advising about, prescribing, or administering medicines. It also helps to clarify why medicines have inconsistent effectiveness or treatment adherence and their effects, side effects, interactions and associated risks can vary and be unpredictable. Table 5.1 summarises and gives some examples.

Ideal medicine	Most medicines
Effective This is when the desired response is achieved by the drug. Medicines are unlikely to be approved unless a body of evidence suggests they are effective. We assume drugs meet their stated purpose or indication, although sometimes they are used outside of this (e.g. off licence).	Research and guidelines show that medicines have variable rates or degrees of effectiveness. For example, warfarin has clearly been shown to achieve the desired effect of thinning blood. However, prescribing it for stroke prevention (in people with atrial fibrillation) has a relatively small measurable impact on that clinical outcome. Its effectiveness varies depending on the severity of the assessed risk of stroke (NICE, 2021a).
Safe A safe drug would produce no ill-effects, even with repeated, excessive doses or long-term use. It is recognised that medicinal preparations can potentially cause harm, so guidance on forms, use and doses aim to reduce risks.	Few drugs are completely safe even when there is adherence to prescribing guidelines. There are variations to the severity of these risks. Common examples include antibiotics which may cause anaphylaxis; chemotherapy drugs which can result in severe neutropenia; or opioid analgesics which can cause potentially fatal respiratory depression. Prescribers need to be able to explain risks, benefits and know where to find accurate information.
Selective The perfect drug would work selectively to cause only the wanted effect. It would target specific areas within the body and act to produce only the desired effect, without causing side effects or adverse drug reactions (ADRs).	It is widely recognised that drugs are not entirely selective as they produce a range of effects, both beneficial and unwanted, and sometimes harmful. Where these are predictable, and short-lasting, they are quantified as side effects (BNF, JFC). Other undesirable or unpredictable effects may be harmful and prevent therapy continuing (adverse drug effects). For example, salbutamol's intended site of action is Beta 2 receptors within the lungs which causes bronchodilation. However, as it is non-selective, it also binds to Beta1 receptors in the heart, which can cause tachycardia or arrhythmias.

(Continued)

Table 5.1   (Continued)

Ideal medicine	Most medicines
Reversible For some drugs it is beneficial to reverse their effect at a selected time (such as anaesthesia). Drugs can potentially cause harm or toxicity and when stopping it is insufficient, it would be 'ideal' to have a reversal agent.	The effects of some drugs can be reversed if needed, but not all. For example, vitamin K can be given to help counteract a warfarin overdose, but there is no equivalent for some of the 'Direct acting oral anticoagulants' (**DOACs**) such as edoxaban (BNF, JFC). This emphasises the importance of a thorough person-centred decision-making process before prescribing or administering any medication considering the risk versus benefit.
Predictable A risk of harm would be reduced if we could accurately predict the impact of a medicine on an individual. The ideal medicine would produce no unexpected actions or effects.	While we can predict the risks linked to some conditions or drug combinations (resulting in contra-indications and cautions), people are individual in their responses, so this is not always possible. In the BNF, side effects are classified as very common or common, uncommon, rare and very rare so it is always good to check. For example, very rare blood clots following certain vaccines may not be predictable, but once known can be considered.
Easy to administer The ideal medicines would be delivered in a form and at time intervals that are suited to the situation or a person's preferences.	While some medicines can be adjusted for convenience, in many cases this doesn't apply. For example, insulin injections may be needed twice a day or simvastatin at night, but other medicines in the morning. Adherence to medicines can also be affected by complicated regimes, particularly if there is little understanding of the reason for these.
Free from interactions The ideal drug has no undesirable interactions with other medicines or diet.	Interactions between drugs can lessen or potentiate the effects. While some interactions can be beneficial, many are unwanted and may cause adverse effects. An example of a beneficial interaction could be the use of two anti-hypertensives that work *synergically*, causing an exaggerated response for people with very high blood pressure. The increased risk of digoxin toxicity with salbutamol is an example of an unwanted interaction.
Cost effective An ideal drug would be affordable and cost effective. Drug costs are significant at around £15 billion per year (NHS Digital, 2020). They are an ever-growing financial outlay as new products are regularly marketed.	As a prescriber, you are normally guided and sometimes limited by what is available via local or national formularies. All NICE guidance includes an economic analysis and if a medicine is not deemed to be cost effective, it will not be supported or available to prescribe, even when it has proven clinical benefit. For instance, a newly developed drug (Orkambi) was proven to be of significant benefit to children with cystic fibrosis but was extremely costly. After several years of lobbying by parents, the Scottish NHS first approved its use, followed by NICE in 2020.

Table 5.1   An ideal medicine vs most medicines

In the absence of ideal or perfect medicines, the aim is for optimal benefits with minimal risks of harm. Alongside your knowledge of the person being prescribed for, familiarity with medicinal products and pharmacology enables you to most effectively achieve this. This section explores routes of administration, before outlining some key points of *pharmacokinetics* and *pharmacodynamics*.

Routes of administration

Medicines can be delivered in a variety of ways to produce local or systemic effects, or occasionally both. **Topical** preparations such as ointments generally produce local effects, although there are exceptions – as, for example, steroidal creams or nasal sprays can also act *systemically*. For drugs to have a *systemic* effect they need to be absorbed into the circulation, with the two main routes referred to as **enteral** or **parenteral**. The oral or enteral route involves transit through the gastro-intestinal (**GI**) **system**, while parenteral is outside the GI tract (Burchum and Rosenthal, 2016). The parenteral route includes topical but is usually associated with injections. These can take a variety of forms such as intravenous, intra-muscular, subcutaneous, spinal, intra-dermal, intrathecal, or intra-articular. Activity 5.2 asks you to think about the various routes of administration and why these are important.

Activity 5.2   Critical thinking

Think about medicines you may have taken or seen given to others.

1. List all the different formulations of medicines that are available and consider why there might be so many different forms.
2. Why might this be important when giving medication advice?

Undertake this activity with your practice assessor or supervisor, or when carrying out an insight visit with a pharmacist.

A brief outline answer is provided at the end of the chapter and it is recommended you continue to add to this from observation in the practice setting and through the discussion to follow. Example administration routes and preparations are outlined in Figure 5.1.

In Activity 5.2, you have considered different forms of medication and the advice that may be required. The selected route of administration will influence a medicine's effectiveness, risks and benefit. For example, intravenous (IV) paracetamol works more quickly than oral preparations and is more appropriate in certain circumstances. While both routes can cause **toxicity**, the oral route is advised as this is the most convenient and reduces some risks associated with intravenous administration (eMC, 2020a, b). **Bioavailability** and route of administration are two key factors which affect a medicine reaching its intended site of action to produce a systemic effect. Bioavailability refers to how much of the drug reaches the systemic circulation from where it can travel to its site of action. Tablets are one of the easiest and most convenient ways to administer medication, but not all medicines are available in tablet form or suitable for everyone. For example, if a person has difficulty swallowing, tablets could cause ulceration if left in the mouth (BNF, JFC).

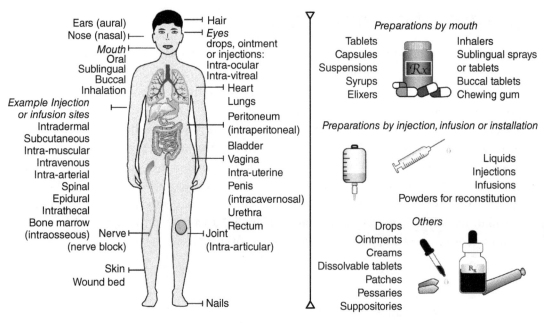

Figure 5.1 Routes of drug administration

Pharmacology and the body

Medicines should be formulated to produce the greatest possible benefit with the least risk of harm, although variables are recognised as per Table 5.1. The extent to which the drug works largely depends on its concentration at the site of action. Numerous mechanisms occur at a cellular and chemical level to prompt action. Revision of anatomy, physiology and biochemistry will help with your awareness of the macro and micro (cellular) processes and how medicines move around the body and produce their effects. The scientific knowledge of how the body works continues to expand, which is reflected in the development of new and more highly specialised or targeted medicines, often trying to address the challenge of getting to the intended sites of action. As most drug actions occur at a cellular level, Figure 5.2 provides a reminder of the different levels of body systems, with a few examples.

The final two levels, cell parts (organelles) and chemistry are not on the table as some of the components are common to all, although there are also variations depending on the type of cell. The two main components of all cells are cytoplasm (the contents) and cytosol (the liquid within the cell). The distinct contents are referred to as organelles and include a nucleus (or several nuclei), ribosomes, mitochondria and various other items. Cytosol is an intracellular solution of nutrients, electrolytes and enzymes. The shape of the cell and some of the contents depend on the type, function and location of the cell. For example, neurons have a sprawling shape with dendrites so they can receive messages from other cells, while pneumocytes in the lungs are flat 'squamous' cells, with few organelles to better facilitate gas exchange. All have a membrane which

Organism (Body)	Organ systems	Organs (examples)	Tissues (examples)	Cells (examples)	Cell Parts (see text)
	Nervous	Brain	Neural tissue	Neuron	
	Cardiovascular	Heart	Heart muscle	Cardiomyocytes	
	Respiratory	Lungs	Alveoli	Pneumocytes	
	GI - Digestive	Small intestine	Villi	Endothelium	
	Endocrine	Pancreas	Exocrine tissues	Acinar cells	
	Renal-urinary	Kidneys	Glomerulus	Mesangial cells	
	Immune	Lymph nodes	Lymphoid tissue	Lymphocytes	
	Integumental	Skin	Epidermis	Melanocytes	
	Muscular	Deltoid	Skeletal muscle	Myofiber	
	Skeletal	Femur	Compact bone	Osteocytes	

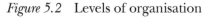

Figure 5.2 Levels of organisation

(illustrations adapted from Ashelford *et al.*, 2019)

envelopes the cell, separating it from the extracellular fluid and regulating what enters and exits. Most drug molecules travel through the cells by **diffusion**, which involves movement from areas of higher concentration to lower concentration. While the rate of diffusion across a cell membrane is mainly determined by gradient (or difference in concentration), the molecule's size, lipid solubility and the area of absorptive surface also affect the rate, or if it can pass through. The chemical and cellular characteristics of molecules are key to pharmacokinetic and pharmacodynamic processes.

Pharmacokinetics: the effect the body has on the drug

Kinetics refer to movement and pharmacokinetic processes refer to the movement of drugs around the body over time. Figure 5.3 broadly shows how the body processes a systemic drug, sometimes in a cyclic way and depending on the route, drug form and various other factors. For most preparations, it is usually broken down into four key stages: *Absorption, Distribution* (pre- and post-liver), *Metabolism* and *Excretion* (or ADME). *Metabolism* (**biotransformation***) and *excretion* together are sometimes referred to as *elimination*.

As can be seen from Figure 5.3, the journey of medicines through the body is not always linear, as, for example, some steps can occur repeatedly in a cycle, such as metabolism through the liver. The way the body processes a drug varies from person to person, and there are many factors that can affect these processes such as the drug's composition, form and dose or the recipient's age and physical condition. Each of these four main processes are considered in more detail in their usual sequence of occurrence.

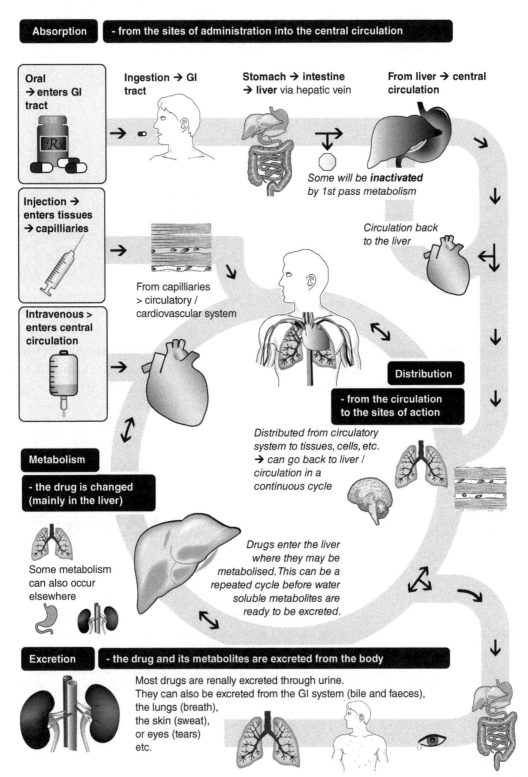

Figure 5.3 The movement of systemic drugs around the body

Absorption

Absorption describes the movement of a drug from the site of administration into the blood, or circulatory system. The site of drug absorption will depend on the route of administration – for example, an oral preparation will be absorbed from the GI tract and an intra-muscular injection from the tissues. *Bioavailability* refers to how much of the administered drug reaches the systemic circulation. This differs depending on the administration route. There is no absorption required for intravenous administration and bioavailability is 100 per cent as it is given directly into the systemic circulation. For other routes bioavailability will be less as some of the drug will be lost during **first-pass metabolism** or absorption. Oral preparations have greatly variable rates which are often expressed as a range. For example, paracetamol bioavailability is 100 per cent for intravenous, ranges from 63–89 per cent for oral administration and 24–98 per cent rectally (Sharma and Mehta, 2014).

Oral drug absorption

Oral administration is the most common and convenient route of drug administration. However, absorption via this route can be complicated and some drugs may not be suitable orally because they are completely inactivated by the defensive action of the gastric acid. For example, insulin is inactivated by gastro-intestinal enzymes so must be given parenterally (BNF, JFC). Oral absorption can also be less effective due to first-pass metabolism. This mechanism aims to protect the body from ingested toxins by filtering them through the liver before they reach the systemic circulation. Oral drugs are primarily absorbed in the small intestine and enter the liver via the hepatic portal vein. Here a proportion of the drug may undergo rapid metabolism before it has a chance to reach the systemic circulation. The higher the rate of first-pass metabolism the lower the bioavailability of the drug, requiring a higher dose. For some drugs such as glyceryl trinitrate, first-pass metabolism is so great following oral administration that it is only effective if given by alternative routes such as sublingual, transdermal, or intravenous. When drugs are developed, their forms and dosages take this into account.

Oral drug absorption can also be altered for other reasons such as gastro-intestinal factors, food and fluid, other medicines, **co-morbidities**, formulation or composition and age. These are discussed in further detail.

- **Gastro-intestinal factors**
  - **Gastric emptying:** an increase in gastric emptying into the small intestine (where absorption mainly occurs) will make the absorption rate quicker. If it is delayed, the delivery of the drug to the intestine is slower, thus reducing the absorption rate and risking it being destroyed by the stomach acid. Gastric emptying time can vary from minutes up to 12 hours and is affected by age. For example, the rate is slower and irregular for infants, while older adults are known to have reduced gastric emptying, thus affecting drug absorption (Burchum *et al.*, 2016).

For drugs (such as aspirin) that are absorbed from the stomach, the slower gastric emptying time will increase its absorption.

- o **Gut motility:** when this is increased there is quicker transit through the GI system, therefore less time for the drug to be in contact with absorptive membranes. For example, when someone has diarrhoea, they may not absorb as much of a drug as usual. Conversely, when motility is slow, the extended transit time means more of the drug could be absorbed.

- o **Gut pH:** The pH varies at points along the GI system, and this can affect the absorption rates of medicines. Some drugs (such as itraconazole or ketoconazole) require a more acidic environment in the gut in order to dissolve and be absorbed. Gastric acid production is lower in infants, until about two years of age, and is also reduced in older adults. Enteric-coated drugs are designed to withstand the environment of the stomach (acids and digestive enzymes like pepsin) so they can proceed to the intestines where their coating is broken down. However, if gastric emptying is delayed, there may be reduction in absorption as the protective coating is broken down in the stomach.

- **Food and fluid:** These can both selectively increase or decrease the absorption rate. For example, some antibiotics are adversely affected by the presence of dairy products (calcium), while fluid can help dissolve medicines and ease passage to the small intestine. Some medicines will specifically need to be taken with or after food whereas others will need to be taken on an empty stomach. This is because the amount of drug absorbed can be affected by the presence of food in the GI tract.

- **Other medication:** Some drugs can alter the absorption of others if taken at the same time. An important example of this is indigestion remedies as they contain heavy metals such as aluminium or calcium which can prevent the absorption of some commonly used antibiotics such as tetracyclines by irreversibly binding to the drug and inactivating it. Antacids can also cause a change in the pH which can increase or decrease the absorption of other drugs.

- **Co-morbidities:** The health of the gastro-intestinal tract can affect absorption so the presence of co-morbidities could affect the rate and amount of drug absorbed. For example, people with a stoma may have altered absorption depending on the site of their stoma. The oral route may not be appropriate in certain conditions which may limit absorption such as vomiting or diarrhoea. There are clear contra-indications where drugs are known to cause gastric irritation or bleeding (such as aspirin) (BNF, JFC), for those who have known gastric ulcers.

- **Formulation and composition:** Various factors related to the composition or formulation can affect absorption rate. For example, liquid preparations or **lipid-soluble** drugs are more readily absorbed, while enteric-coated drugs are slower. Some drug formulations are designed to alter the rate of absorption to give a prolonged effect such as modified release tablets or capsules. Enteric-coated drugs have a coating, while modified release preparations consist of many small parts of the drug with coatings that break down at different rates.

- **Age:** As outlined above, extremes of age can affect a person's ability to absorb medications orally in various ways due to delayed gut motility, increased gut pH and reduced absorptive surface areas. Some preparations, such as ibuprofen, are cautioned due to remaining in the stomach longer, being broken down and causing irritation from direct contact with the mucosa or stomach lining.

Parenteral drug absorption

While oral administration is the most common and convenient route, for various reasons parenteral may be necessary or preferred. Some medicines are clearly unsuitable for oral delivery as they are inactivated through digestive enzymes or first-pass metabolism, while there are several other reasons to administer parenterally. For example, in emergency situations such as anaphylaxis where an immediate effect is required, preparations such as adrenaline are the standard treatment (BNF, JFC). Some drugs have a narrow margin between effective and toxic, so drug blood levels need to be tightly controlled. Some cytotoxic preparations such as platinum-based cisplatin have anti-cancer activity but can damage other tissues including skin, soft tissue or mucous membranes, so are only administered by infusion (BNF, JFC). Some drugs are rapidly absorbed, leading to elevated plasma drug concentration beyond their therapeutic level causing toxicity, therefore it may be preferable to give an injection such as a depot where the drug is released slowly into the blood stream from fat or muscle. A further reason for parenteral administration may be in people who are unable to take oral preparations – for example, if they are vomiting, unconscious, or lack capacity to understand instructions.

Absorption for medicines administered *parenterally* ranges from immediate to more gradual dependent on the injection site, perfusion, proximity to the circulatory system and properties of solution; an oily base will improve absorption. For example, intravenous administration results in immediate 100 per cent *bioavailability* as it bypasses any *absorption* barriers such as first-pass metabolism. Advantages to this route include being able to use irritants (e.g. chemotherapy medicines) as when given with IV fluid they are rapidly diluted in the bloodstream. Parenteral routes such as intradermal injections diffuse more slowly into the local capillaries, while this is slightly quicker for subcutaneous injections. The condition of tissues at the site is significant, as, for example, people with long-term diabetes who don't sufficiently rotate their injection sites can develop areas where the insulin is inadequately absorbed. Intra-muscular injections are reasonably fast to absorb due to the rich supply of blood to muscle tissue, although these too can be affected by local tissue damage. Bioavailability can be influenced in other ways – for example, with adrenaline auto-injectors it is potentially affected by the formulation as well as the propulsive force of the device and needle length (BNF, JFC).

There are many topical routes for local effect, such as the skin, mouth, eyes, ears, nose, or nails. Drugs applied to the skin and some of the mucous membranes are normally slower to act systemically than either parenteral or oral, although this is dependent on access to the vascular system and the preparation. For example, if a topical ointment is applied to broken skin, or covered by an occlusive dressing, this can increase systemic absorption (due to being closer to the capillaries or creating a warmer environment). Some forms of topical agents such as glyceryl trinitrate (BNF, JFC) are specifically formulated for transdermal absorption providing rapid absorption into the systemic circulation. Systemic absorption of rectal and sublingual preparations can be quite rapid because of the vascularity of those areas. Nasal preparations can work both locally and systemically, with varying degrees of rapidity. Minimal systemic effects result from installation into the ears such as olive oil, although the use of almond oil ear drops is contra-indicated due to risks for people with nut allergies (BNF, JFC). Absorption from the eyes depends on the preparation – for example, whether drops or ointment – while intra-ocular or intra-vitreous injections would be most rapid.

Inhaled drugs can also work both locally and systemically. For example, the main actions of asthma preparations are in the lungs, but some side effects, such as tachycardia, are due to their systemic absorption and action on receptors in the heart. With the use of inhaled steroids, rinsing the mouth with water is recommended following use to prevent oral fungal infections such as candidiasis arising. Other inhalational agents such as anaesthetics are intentionally used for their systemic effects and are rapidly absorbed. Some conditions require drugs to be given by direct injection into a specific site – for example, into the heart, spine, nerves, bone marrow or joints. These preparations have unique characteristics and are intended for local action, although some may also be absorbed into the circulatory system and produce systemic effects.

The importance of correct administration route and formulation cannot be overstated. For example, errors have been made whereby drugs intended for intravenous administration were given spinally, or oral solutions given intravenously, with devastating effects. In one instance, potassium permanganate tablets were administered orally instead of being dissolved in water for external use, with fatal consequences. There are also cautions associated with administering medications in ways not intended or licensed. For example, opening a capsule or crushing an enteric-coated medicine to use in a feeding tube can alter the way a medicine works with a risk of causing side effects (UKMi, 2020).

This section looked at the absorption, which is the first stage in the pharmacokinetic process of ADME. Absorption refers to the movement of a drug into the systemic circulation. Activity 5.3 asks you to apply this to the example case study.

Activity 5.3   Critical thinking

Considering our scenario of Madiba and the available forms of ibuprofen.

1. What is the site of absorption for each form?
2. What factors might affect the absorption of the different forms?

An outline answer is provided at the end of the chapter.

Now that you have critically considered the scenario with Madiba in relation to drug absorption, we can explore the next ADME stage of *Distribution*. Where absorption was primarily concerned with the drug getting into the cardiovascular system, drug distribution is the movement of the drug out of that system and to the intended sites of action.

Drug distribution

Distribution is the process in which the drug molecule is transported from the site of absorption to the target site of action, such as cell receptors. The drug needs to reach its intended site of action to achieve any effect. This primarily means travelling from the systemic circulation to the various tissues and cells. All blood vessels contain a layer of endothelial cells, while the larger arteries and veins also have layers of smooth muscle cells and connective tissues. The endothelium performs several roles including acting as a barrier. Capillaries consist of a single layer of endothelial cells, along with a basal lamina and pericytes (Alberts *et al.*, 2002). Figures 5.4 and 5.5 show the cells of blood vessels and capillaries where, given the right conditions, drug molecules can enter or exit.

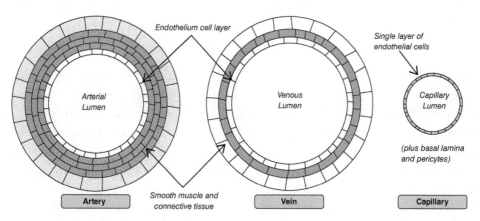

Figure 5.4   Blood vessel and capillary walls

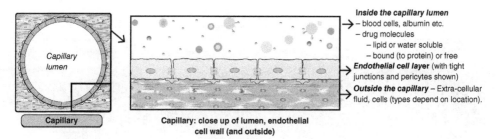

Figure 5.5   Capillary endothelium

While capillaries and their cell membranes help regulate what can enter and exit the circulatory system, several other factors influence the movement of drug molecules throughout the body. Some of the influences on drug distribution are outlined, including:

the drug's ability to move into the tissues and cells (movement to the tissues); the blood brain and placental barriers; blood flow/supply; storage sites; and protein binding.

Influences on drug distribution

Movement to the tissues: Drugs leave the bloodstream at capillary beds and need to pass through the cell membranes. Cell membranes regulate the concentration of substances inside the cell such as nutrients (sugar, amino acids), ions (calcium, potassium, etc.) and waste products, such as carbon dioxide. As illustrated in Figure 5.6, cell membranes have a phospholipid bilayer, interspersed with various forms of protein and allow small non-polar molecules such as oxygen, alcohol and other lipids to move through. Lipid-soluble drug molecules (the majority) can easily pass through this layer of fatty acids, but **water-soluble** drugs have more difficulty. Similarly, larger molecule drugs and those bound to a large molecule (e.g. protein) are unable to pass through the capillary wall (see *protein binding*). An example drug that has difficulty passing is vitamin B12 as it requires intrinsic factor for transport across the cell walls. People who lack intrinsic factor will need injections to ensure they obtain sufficient B12.

Most drugs (estimated at over 90 per cent) readily move through the cells via diffusion. Several alternative ways of getting to the bloodstream and from there to the sites of action have been identified as illustrated in Figure 5.7.

Blood brain barrier: This refers to the distinctive anatomy of capillaries and cells in the central nervous system. Unlike other capillaries, the ones in the blood brain barrier contain elaborate close-knit junctions in the cell walls. These tight-knit endothelial cells along with astrocyte cells create a barrier to the brain or cerebrospinal fluid, constraining the passage of molecules. When small molecules do diffuse through the cell membranes, efflux transport proteins can pump them back out, further limiting access to the brain which is a recognised challenge for developing effective drugs to reach the central nervous system. Only *lipid-soluble* drugs such as diazepam (eMC, 2019) or those with an effective transport system can cross through the cell walls to reach sites of action.

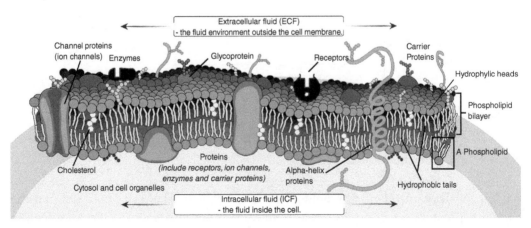

Figure 5.6   Cell membrane

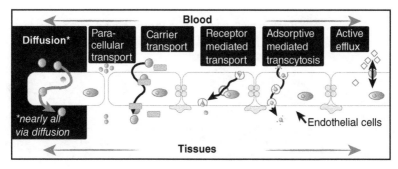

Figure 5.7   Example methods of cell transport

(adapted from a figure in Georgieva *et al.*, 2014)

The blood brain barrier is less developed at birth so infants are more vulnerable to the effects of drugs that can cross this barrier. The mechanisms around drug movement across the body's natural barriers are not all fully understood and drug development research continues to examine proposed pathways (Georgieva *et al.*, 2014).

Placental barrier: Foetal capillaries have a layer of protection that enables only lipid-soluble, non-ionised, or small molecule compounds to pass from mother to child. The placental membrane contains a layer of cells to protect the foetal capillaries but is not an absolute barrier as drug molecules can readily pass from the maternal bloodstream into the blood of the foetus. This includes many that can cause serious harm, such as opioids. As there is such a risk, nurses are advised against prescribing for pregnant women if it is for a pregnancy-related problem, and in most instances should seek expert advice (RCN, 2021a).

Blood supply: The rate of drug delivery to a particular tissue is determined by blood flow to that tissue. Most tissues are well perfused and for those with a good blood supply (e.g. major organs) distribution is usually rapid. However, areas with poor blood supply such as extremities or bone tissue may have poor drug distribution resulting in slower or reduced delivery to the sites of action. Factors such as the person's activity levels, the presence of vascular disease or reduced heart function, or tissue temperature can affect distribution to the extremities or muscles.

Storage sites: Some lipid-soluble drugs may accumulate in fat tissue and not be released or metabolised until a later time, leading to extended half-lives and side effects. Medicines that are bound to calcium may collect in calcium-rich places such as teeth or bones. An example of this is tetracycline which can cause tooth discolouration as a known side effect in children under eight years of age or in children born after use by their pregnant mothers (BNF, JFC).

Protein binding: Drugs form reversible bonds with protein in the blood (mainly albumin). Albumin is such a large molecule it is confined to the bloodstream (Figure 5.8). Drug–protein binding occurs to differing extents depending on the drug's affinity for the proteins (lipid-soluble drugs have higher affinity over water-soluble drugs). Because a

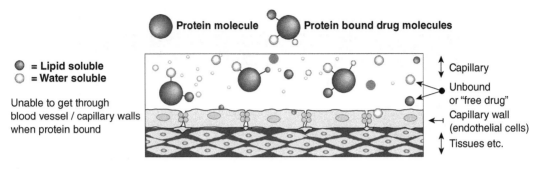

Figure 5.8 Protein binding

protein-bound drug is unable to leave the bloodstream, it cannot have any pharmacological effect so is inactive in the bound state. It is only the unbound drug or *'free drug'* that can be distributed into cells, tissues or other site of action to have an effect. As protein-bound drug molecules cannot reach their sites of action or move on to the stages of metabolism and excretion, the distribution phase is extended which increases the drug's **half-life**.

Although not to scale, Figure 5.8 provides an illustration of the relative size of an albumin molecule with free and bound drug molecules. If albumin (or other protein) molecules levels are reduced in the blood, which can happen due to medical conditions such as liver disease, there will be more 'free' or unbound drug available to act. In addition to a prolonged distribution phase, greater protein binding can increase the risk of *drug interactions* and *adverse events*. Because binding is non-specific, drug molecules will compete for binding sites on plasma proteins. Drugs considered to be 'highly protein bound' are more susceptible to drug interactions because one drug can displace another leading to changes in the amount of free drug. This is important when starting a new drug – for example, warfarin is approximately 99 per cent bound to plasma proteins (eMC, 2017). If another highly protein-bound drug, such as amoxicillin (eMC, 2020) or aspirin is started, it can compete and displace the warfarin creating an increase in the amount of free warfarin. In this instance, more of the warfarin molecules are free to act, causing a higher INR (International Normalised Ratio) and greater risk of bleeding. The BNF (JFC) identifies this as a known adverse reaction/ interaction, but the effect varies and is potentially fatal. Interactions are shown in the BNF, so if a new drug is to be added, this should always be checked.

Protein binding: who is at risk?

It is important to consider protein binding when prescribing for people vulnerable to lower albumin levels (**hypoalbuminaemia**) as these are often whom we are prescribing for: people who are older, acutely ill, malnourished, or with multi-morbidities. Albumin is the most common plasma protein, synthesised in the liver, and serves many important functions (Moman *et al.*, 2020). Some of these include maintaining pressure balance to prevent fluids from leaking into the extravascular spaces, storing, binding and carrying fatty acids, compounds or hormones or binding to compounds such as drugs to reduce toxicity (Gounden *et al.*, 2020). Clinically, albumin levels can be measured as a marker of a person's nutritional status (Yuwen *et al.*, 2017).

Hypoalbuminaemia can be caused by reduced production (liver disease) or its loss due to nutritional deficiency, nephrotic syndrome, chronic kidney disease, other chronic diseases, extravascular losses (e.g. due to sepsis or burns), critical illness or cardiac failure (Gounden *et al.*, 2020). As a prescriber, we need to be aware of groups at higher risk, including older people, those with acute illnesses (such as sepsis), or chronic conditions, particularly liver disease. It is also useful to be alert to the symptoms such as peripheral (pitting), central or generalised oedema, fatigue and excessive weakness or features of the primary disease.

We have looked at protein binding and the risks of low protein. Activity 5.4 asks you to critically think about what this might mean for the distribution of ibuprofen.

Activity 5.4   Critical thinking

Considering our scenario with Madiba and the distribution of ibuprofen:

1.   Is ibuprofen highly protein bound?
2.   Given her age, what might you assess for if several of her medications were highly protein bound?

An outline answer is provided at the end of the chapter.

Now that you have considered the scenario with Madiba's ibuprofen in relation to distribution the next ADME stage, metabolism, can be explored. Distribution was concerned with the drug getting from the vascular system to the intended sites of action. Metabolism occurs mainly within the liver, whose job it is to protect the body from toxins, although it can also occur in a variety of places along the medication's journey.

Metabolism

Drug metabolism is the process by which the chemical composition of a drug molecule is modified or altered, usually in the liver. Also referred to as *biotransformation*, it involves several processes which result in alteration of the original compound. The main aim is to create a more water-soluble **metabolite** which is inactive and can be excreted. Other outcomes of drug metabolism can include drug *inactivation*, increased or decreased therapeutic action, activation of '**prodrugs**' and increased or decreased *drug toxicity* (Table 5.2). The products of metabolism (metabolites) usually have their

Effect	Notes	Examples
Preparation for renal excretion	Converts *lipid-soluble* drugs into more *water-soluble* forms that are able to be excreted	Many drugs: some would take years to excrete without this change
Inactivation	Transformation of pharmacologically active drugs into an inactive form	Prednisolone is metabolised into an inactive metabolite
Activation of 'prodrugs'	A prodrug is pharmacologically inactive in its administered form. Metabolism converts the drug to its active state	Converts ramipril to ramiprilat. Converts codeine phosphate to morphine and norcodeine, with the analgesic effect mainly due to its conversion to morphine
Increased drug action	The effectiveness of some drugs is increased when metabolism converts them to a different compound(s)	Amitriptyline inhibits the uptake of noradrenaline and serotonin. Its most active metabolite is nortriptyline which is a more potent inhibitor of noradrenaline than of serotonin uptake (eMc, 2021a)
Increased or decreased toxicity	Metabolism converts some drugs into inactive forms, so decreases toxicity. For some drugs, the risk of toxic effects is increased through converting relatively safe compounds into more toxic forms	Paracetamol produces a metabolite (N-acetyl-p-benzoquinoneimine) which is usually detoxified by the liver. This metabolite can cause toxicity and liver injury particularly for at risk populations (such as young children, people with liver disease, chronic alcoholism, chronic malnutrition or receiving enzyme inducers). Overdosing may be fatal in these cases (eMC, 2020)

Table 5.2 Potential effects of metabolism

pharmacological activity removed and are more easily excreted than the original drug. For some drugs, the process produces an active form known as an **active metabolite** which can cause either a desired therapeutic effect or an undesirable *adverse effect*.

Drugs can be metabolised by **Phase 1** or **Phase 2** *reactions*. Phase 1 reactions often involve the **cytochrome P450 (CYP450)** family of **enzymes** found in the liver. They often bio-transform the drug to a more manageable metabolite. These enzymes may be affected by drugs causing increased activation or inhibition.

Some drugs undergo only Phase 1 or Phase 2 reactions.

Phase 1 reactions:

* include: oxidation, reduction and hydrolysis;
* usually form more reactive products, sometimes toxic;
* often involve mixed function oxidase system in which cytochrome P450 plays a key role.

Phase 2 reactions:

* include: conjugation;
* usually form inactive, **polar** and readily excretable products through the kidneys or bile.

	Actions/effects	Examples *(these lists are not exhaustive)*
Enzyme inducer	Speeds up drug metabolism of affected drugs Lowers plasma concentration of affected drug Potential for reduced effectiveness	Phenytoin, Phenobarbitone, Carbamazepine, Rifampicin, Griseofulvin, chronic alcohol intake, smoking
Enzyme inhibitor	Slows down drug metabolism of affected drugs Increases plasma concentration of affected drug Potential for toxicity, a pronounced effect and/or increased adverse drug reactions	Erythromycin, Ciprofloxacin, Metronidazole, Chloramphenicol, Sulphonamides, acute alcohol, Allopurinol, Phenylbutazone, Isoniazid, oral contraceptives, Sodium valproate, Cimetidine, Omeprazole, calcium channel blockers, Amiodarone, Dextropropoxyphene, Fluconazole

Table 5.3   Enzyme inducers and inibitors

Phase 2 reactions involves conjugation (normally addition of a water molecule) of Phase 1 metabolites which are not yet water soluble and therefore ready for excretion by the kidney.

Some drugs are known as **enzyme inducers** (Table 5.3); they have the ability to speed up the enzyme reactions, therefore speeding up the metabolism of other drugs metabolised by these enzymes. Conversely some drugs are known as **enzyme inhibitors** which slow down enzyme reactions, and therefore slow down drugs metabolised by this pathway.

Influences on drug metabolism

Just like other processes, there are numerous factors which can affect or alter metabolism. As most metabolism occurs in the liver, factors affecting its function such as the extremes of age or liver failure can have a significant impact.

Age: Liver function varies throughout the life span. Therefore, metabolism can alter depending on the person's age. For example, infants have reduced ability to metabolise drugs since their liver is immature and has not yet developed to full capacity. Age-related decline in liver function is commonly found in older people. Other effects of ageing on metabolism include a reduction in hepatic blood flow leading to reduced first-pass metabolism, delayed production and elimination of active metabolites as liver enzyme systems decrease and an increased risk of the toxic effects of the drug. Although metabolism is primarily within the liver, it can also occur in lungs, kidneys, intestines and blood, so there can be several ways in which metabolism can be compromised at the extremes of age. It is recognised that a drug may need to be stopped or dosages may need to be adjusted down to prevent the risks of drug toxicity. For example, reports suggest paracetamol overdose is linked to lower-weight older adults not having doses correctly adjusted for weight (HSIB, 2021a). Similarly, HSIB, (2021b) has found drug errors in children linked to lack of attention to required adjustments based on the child's weight.

First-pass effect: This normally refers to the rapid *inactivation* of drugs before they reach the systemic circulation. This is most often oral drugs metabolised by the liver, but it can also occur in other tissues capable of metabolism such as the GI tract, lungs, or vascular system. Once oral medicines are absorbed, drug molecules are carried from the stomach or small intestine directly to the liver via the hepatic portal vein. Some drugs can be completely inactivated in their first pass through the liver, while others have a proportion of the drug removed before it can enter the systemic circulation. The drug's effect and further metabolism alter in line with how much of it is left after undergoing first-pass metabolism. For example, the intravenous dose of Propranolol is 1mg, but if given orally the equivalent is 40mg (BNF, JFC).

Genetics: Due to differences such as enzyme systems, genetics may play a role in the rate in which an individual can metabolise certain drugs. For example, some people metabolise codeine rapidly while others metabolise it slowly or not at all; this could lead to increased plasma drug levels of metabolites and side effects, or no therapeutic effect respectively.

Gender: There is some suggestion that women and men differ in the metabolism of certain drugs, and this is linked to the differences in hormones. Pharmacokinetics in women is affected by lower body weight, slower gastro-intestinal motility, less intestinal enzymatic activity and slower glomerular filtration rate.

Ethnicity: There have been differences identified in relation to specific enzymes or compounds needs for metabolism. For example, glucose-6-phosphate dehydrogenase **(G6PD) deficiency** is an inherited condition most prevalent in people originating in the Mediterranean region, sub-Saharan Africa, Asia and the Middle East. This deficiency affects the metabolism of several common medicines such as nitrofurantoin and silver sulfadiazine dressings. These are contra-indicated for anyone with this deficiency, while the BNF (JFC) notes cautions for other drugs such as sulfonylureas, quinolone antibiotics and aspirin.

Nutritional status: In people who are undernourished, cofactors required for metabolism may be deficient. For example, people with cachexia have been shown to poorly metabolise oxycodone, due to a deficiency in liver enzymes (CYP2D6 and CYP3A) (Naito *et al.*, 2012).

Competition between drugs: When two or more drugs use the same metabolic pathway, they may compete for metabolism. The effect of this can be a decrease in how quickly one or both are metabolised, and impact on half-life. This raises potential for extended effects and side effects. Where the metabolism of a drug is reduced (in this or other ways), potentially unsafe accumulation can occur.

Disease: While most of metabolism takes place in the liver, the hepatic reserve is large so liver disease must be severe before major changes in drug metabolism occur (BNF, JFC).

Where there is severe hepatic impairment (acute or chronic), this is likely to have an effect on the rate of metabolism of some drugs and therefore drugs may need to be stopped, or the dose adjusted. The BNF (JFC) suggests it isn't possible to predict the extent to which the metabolism of a particular drug may be impaired, making this risk difficult to accurately assess. Other conditions can impact upon the rate of metabolism, including those that reduce hepatic blood flow, such as heart failure, shock or sepsis.

Renal disease: Where metabolism takes place in the kidneys, renal impairment may require other forms to be prescribed. For example, alfacalcidol (the active form) in place of Vitamin D that requires transformation to its active parts (BNF, JFC). There is also a risk of some products of metabolism collecting in the plasma due to renal impairment.

Tolerance: When some drugs are given repeatedly, metabolism becomes more effective, leaving less of the active substance, thereby requiring larger doses. This ability to deactivate the drug more swiftly is one of the processes leading to tolerance. Drug tolerance can pose a problem with medicines affecting the central nervous system such as analgesia and has implications for prescribing. For example, in people requiring post-surgical pain relief who are opioid-dependent, a non-standard dose adjustment will be needed for the same therapeutic effect to be achieved. In relation to dependency, there have been new safety recommendations issued following a review of the risks of dependence and addiction associated with prolonged use (more than three months) of opioids for non-malignant pain (BNF, JFC). It can take several months for receptor numbers to return to pre-drug levels.

We have provided an overview of some of the key features of drug metabolism. Activity 5.5 enables you to apply some of these principles with the BNF (JFC) and eMC as recommended information sources.

Activity 5.5   Critical thinking

The herbal remedy St John's wort is available to purchase for the treatment of mild depression and known to be an enzyme inducer.

1. Describe what the phrase 'enzyme inducer' means in terms of metabolism.
2. With reference to BNF interactions for St John's wort, identify three drugs that interact with St John's wort and what the effect is.
3. Thinking to our scenario with Madiba, would it be a problem for him to take ibuprofen if he decided to take St John's wort?

An outline answer is provided at the end of the chapter.

Now that you have critically considered the principles of metabolism, the next ADME stage concerns the removal of the drug from the body, or *excretion.*

Excretion

The main site of drug excretion is the kidneys via the urine. Therefore, kidney function plays a significant part in how drugs are excreted from the body. Other sites where drugs and metabolites can be excreted include from the liver (through bile and faeces), through sweat, saliva, tears, exhaled breathe and breastmilk. The extent to which drugs pass into these secretions can vary. Renal drug excretion is known to have three main processes: **glomerular filtration**, **passive tubular reabsorption** and **active tubular secretion.**

Drug filtration occurs in the renal capillaries where drug molecules move from the blood into the urine tubules. Protein-bound molecules are too large to get through so remain in the blood. In the next step, passive tubular reabsorption, lipid-soluble drug molecules can be reabsorbed into the blood, whereas drugs that aren't lipid soluble remain in the urine to be excreted. The third step, active tubular secretion, involves active transport systems in the kidney tubules along with P-glycoprotein, which can pump a variety of drugs into the urine for excretion. As with other processes, there are numerous factors that can affect drug excretion. These include kidney function, age, the water solubility and half-life of the drug, urine pH and competition between drugs; these are explained further.

Kidney function: Renal excretion serves to limit the duration of action of many drugs. How well the kidneys are working can affect how quickly the drug acts, for how long, the intensity of the drug response and how much of a drug is excreted. Changes in kidney function can alter drug response and its effect. If kidney function declines, either suddenly due to an acute kidney injury or over time due to chronic kidney disease, the amount of drug excretion may reduce. This can lead to drug toxicity if the drug is continued, or if dose adjustments are not made.

Age: Renal function varies with age. Renal function of the very young such as neonates is not developed like that of an adult, so they excrete drugs differently. With ageing there is loss of nephrons, typically starting after the age of 40, and subsequent decline in kidney function especially after age of 65. Older people are likely to have a reduced kidney function putting them at more risk of adverse drug reactions and toxicity. Therefore, renal function needs to be considered when dosing medication and for monitoring after it has been prescribed.

Water solubility of the drug: Drugs that are water soluble are more likely to be excreted unchanged along with water-soluble metabolites. Adjustments to dosage may be more significant when someone has a poor renal function, particularly for drugs with a narrow therapeutic index.

Half-life: The half-life of a drug refers to the time it takes for the plasma concentration of the drug to be reduced by half. This could be affected by how well the kidneys excrete the drug. For example, an older person with a declining renal function may take longer to clear the drug (have a longer half-life) than a healthy adult. Often drugs that have a shorter half-life are selected for use in older people for this reason and are associated with less prolonged adverse drug reactions.

Urine pH: Passive tubular reabsorption is limited to lipid-soluble compounds. Urinary pH can be altered to decrease passive reabsorption back into the blood, thereby speeding up its excretion. An example of this is treatment of aspirin poisoning, where the BNF (JFC) advises that within certain parameters intravenous sodium bicarbonate may be given to enhance urinary salicylate excretion (aiming for an optimum urinary pH of 7.5–8.5).

Competition between drugs: As with metabolism, there may be competition between drugs for access to the active tubular transport processes. This can result in a prolongation of the effects of drugs that normally undergo rapid renal excretion when there is another drug competing on the same transport system.

This section has discussed some of the key points around drug excretion, which we explore further in the case scenario with Madiba and ibuprofen.

Case scenario

Madiba continues to take his ibuprofen but decides to increase the dose because he is still in pain. He is now taking up to 1.2g each day in divided doses and becomes unwell, with diarrhoea and vomiting over two days. He is eating and drinking very little. However, he continues to take ibuprofen as he feels it is important for his joint pain. Madiba is found to have an acute kidney injury and his renal function suddenly declines rapidly.

Activity 5.6 asks you to apply the principles to identify a potential risk in Madiba's case.

Activity 5.6   Critical thinking

Using the information supplied in the case study:

- discuss the factors that may affect how he excretes the ibuprofen;
- discuss what effect this will have on the excretion of ibuprofen;
- what advice would you give about his ibuprofen while he is unwell?

An outline answer is provided at the end of the chapter.

Activity 5.6 asked you to consider some of the implications of taking a medicine that can affect renal function. This was used to illustrate the importance of always checking prior to prescribing and as a part of advice and ongoing monitoring. Excretion and elimination are seen as the final stage in pharmacokinetics (ADME) or the effect the body has on medicines as they move through the body. We will now look at pharmacodynamics, or the effects medicines have on the body.

Pharmacodynamics

Pharmacodynamics is defined as the effect the drug has on the body. There are several main ways in which drugs produce an effect, such as acting on receptors, enzymes, ion channels, carrier/transporters and on organisms, or working in a non-specific way. Each of these are described with examples provided. The most common way systemic drugs work is when they act on a receptor site. Most receptors are a form of proteins, with one type (the G protein-coupled receptors or GPCRs) being the most studied and prevalent drug targets. Alongside receptors, other drug targets include ion channels, enzymes and transporters. Figure 5.9 provides an illustration of these before they are explained in more depth.

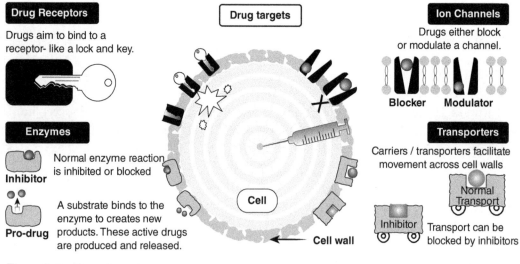

Figure 5.9   Drug targets

Drug receptors

Receptors are found in the cell membrane and cause a response within the cell when they are activated. There are many types of receptors, depending on location; they are effective targets for drugs because action can either be activated (agonised) or blocked (antagonised) (see Figure 5.10).

- **Antagonist**: A drug which blocks a receptor and stops a reaction occurring is known as an antagonist or a blocker. Well-known antagonists include histamine H2-receptor (found in the stomach), antagonists such as ranitidine or antihistamines that suppress allergy symptoms by binding to H1 receptors (found in the nasal passages) for histamine.
- **Agonist**: A drug which stimulates or activates a receptor is known as an agonist. Binding to receptors in this way replicates the body's own mechanisms. Many medicines work in this way; a commonly prescribed example is the beta$_2$ agonist salbutamol (BNF, JFC).
- **Partial agonists**: Some drugs bind to a receptor but produce a lesser effect than a full agonist or have more than one action. For example, most beta-blockers such as atenolol are just antagonists, but a few of them such as buprenorphine also have an ability to act as a partial agonist (BNF, JFC). Intrinsic sympathomimetic activity (ISA, partial agonist activity) represents the capacity of beta-blockers to stimulate as well as to block adrenergic receptors.

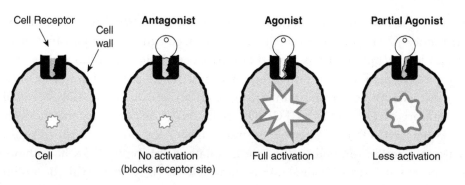

Figure 5.10 Effects on receptor sites

Ion channels

Ion channels are proteins within the cell membrane that form openings enabling the flow of ions. These channels are essential for the electrical signals prompting bodily functions such as electrolyte balance, muscle contraction, neurotransmitter release, hormone secretion, blood pressure, etc. There are hundreds of different ion channels that are often grouped according to the type of 'gate' or opening mechanism. The gates open intermittently in response to specific conditions in the membrane such as a change in electrical membrane potential (voltage-gated channels) or the binding of a neurotransmitter such as adrenaline (ligand-gated channels) (Alberts *et al.*, 2002). Varying types and example medicines are outlined below and seen in Figure 5.10.

- *Voltage-gated ion channels* (VGICs): These open or close in response to changes in the electrical polarity of the cell membrane. There are separate channels for each of the major ions, such as sodium (Na+), potassium (K+), Calcium (Ca+) and Chloride (Cl-). Examples include calcium channel blocking drugs such as amlodipine (BNF, JFC).

- *Ligand-gated ion channels* (LGICs): A **ligand** is a molecule or ion that binds to a channel receptor to trigger a change. These channels enable the quick synaptic transmission in the nervous system and at the somatic neuromuscular junction (IUPHAR, 2021). Example receptors include nicotinic acetylcholine (nAch) or GABA receptors.
- *Other*: Further examples of ion channel types include non-selective, sodium leak or aquaporins (or water channels). This family of chloride channels allow rapid water movement which is vital for processes such as homeostasis, urinary concentration, brain function and skin hydration. An example aquaporin is the cystic fibrosis transmembrane conductance regulator (CFTR) which is present at the surface of epithelial cells in multiple organs. In some people with cystic fibrosis there is defective channel gating. Medicines have been developed to act directly to improve cellular processing and facilitate increased chloride transport by potentiating the channel-open probability (or gating) of the CFTR protein at the cell surface (eMC, 2021c).

Enzymes

Enzymes in the body are important proteins that speed up (catalyse) reactions. Without the presence of enzymes the reactions do not occur and the usual functions of the body can be disrupted. Drugs have therefore been designed to block these enzymes and prevent an action from occurring, or they will mimic the enzymes to initiate an action. An example of an inhibiting drug is ibuprofen which is a non-steroidal anti-inflammatory drug (NSAID) (JFC). Drugs in this class block an enzyme known as cyclooxygenase (COX). COX enzyme is required for the process in which prostaglandins are released in the body causing inflammation. Inhibiting COX has other effects such as potential gastro-intestinal events, although the risk is lower with ibuprofen compared with NSAIDs that are non-selective (BNF, JFC).

Cell transporters/carriers

Cell transporters are found in some cell membranes and facilitate the transport of ions in and out of the cell. The transfer of ions is often a trigger for a chemical reaction to occur within the cell causing an effect. Therefore, some drugs will block cell transporters and block these reactions. An example is the blockage of transporters into the nerve cells, known as neurotransmitters. Tricyclic antidepressants inhibit the neurotransmitter noradrenaline (BNF, JFC).

Organisms

Some drugs are designed to specifically target the cells of invading organisms rather than acting on human cells. This includes antibiotics, antifungals, antivirals and anthelmintics. Within the category of antibacterials, there are different mechanisms of action such as interfering with the bacterial cell wall, or the synthesis of bacterial cell protein or with the replication of their DNA. The structure of targets for antibiotic action, such as the penicillin binding proteins, vary between antibiotics. Different antibiotics have affinities for the various targets. For example, cephalosporins cannot interact with the penicillin binding proteins in enterococci. Glycopeptides such as vancomycin are only active against gram-positive organisms as they cannot penetrate the outer lipo-polysaccharide layer of gram-negative organisms, which gram-positive organisms do not have. Biofilms have been found to be particularly resistant to antibiotics and it is thought that this may be at least partially due to efflux pumps, which send the drug molecules back out of the cells. Evidence of this has been found in several resistant microorganisms such as E-coli and pseudomonas aeruginosa (Soto, 2013) but the mechanism is still poorly understood and research continues into efflux pump inhibitors to help address resistance.

Non-specific actions

Some medication does not act specifically on cells and is therapeutic due to non-specific action. Examples include:

- *antacids*: neutralise stomach acid to prevent or treat heartburn or indigestion;
- *alginates*: form a raft in the stomach to prevent or treat heartburn;
- *bulk forming or osmotic laxatives*: draw fluid into the large bowel to treat constipation;
- *emollients*: trap moisture and aid skin hydration by covering the outer layer of the skin with a greasy film as a barrier to further water loss;
- *cytotoxics*: these drugs work by destroying cells or inhibiting their growth, being toxic to cells. Their anti-cancer activity is achieved in a variety of ways, such as attacking cell membranes causing lysis, or preventing cell division. This can also damage normal tissue and most cytotoxic drugs are teratogenic (BNF, JFC). Chemotherapy may intend to cure, to prolong life or to palliate symptoms. Cytotoxic drugs all cause side effects so there needs to be a balance between the risks associated with toxicity and the likely benefits;
- *anaesthetics*: the precise mechanisms of action are not fully known but anaesthetics broadly work by preventing nerves from sending signals to the brain.

This section outlined some examples of the many ways in which drugs work to produce actions. This can be imperfect so their effect can be inexact, undesirable, and sometimes unpredictable. The next section outlines some of these adverse effects.

Adverse drug reactions

Any drug can produce unwanted or unexpected adverse effects (BNF, JFC). These are normally identified as Type A or Type B adverse drug reactions (ADR), although other types have also been recognised.

Type A (Augmented) ADRs: Some side effects of drugs are predictable because of how the drug works and how it affects the bodily system. The effect is an exaggeration of the action of the drug. This type of reaction, known as Type A reactions, is usually common and manageable by stopping the medication, lowering the dose or taking no action as it may lessen in effect over a few weeks. An example of this type of reaction may be diarrhoea caused by laxative use.

Type B (Bizarre) ADRs: Some side effects are rare and often unrelated to how the drug works. They occur in some people but not in others which makes them 'bizarre' and difficult to predict. These rarer adverse events may be associated with a higher risk of morbidity or mortality. Due to the risk they usually result in the drug being immediately stopped. An example of this type of adverse event is anaphylaxis caused by penicillins.

Other types of ADRs: There are further ADRs which can be classified as *C (continuing)*, *D (delayed)* or *E (end of dose)*. Continuing are reactions that continue for a very long time (MHRA, 2015). An example could be tardive dyskinesia caused by some anti-psychotic medicines. D (delayed) reactions can appear after several weeks or months of use, while E (end of use) adverse effects are withdrawal reactions. An example of this can be anxiety, dizziness, fatigue, sleep disturbances, etc. commonly linked to abrupt withdrawal or dose reduction of Sertraline (BNF, JFC).

Advice regarding adverse effects

It is important to refer people to the patient information leaflet (**PIL**) and to explain the risk of common or significant adverse effects and what action to take if they occur. PILs are available for each preparation on Medicines.org/eMC. Sometimes another drug may be required to treat the side effects of one being taken. The BNF (JFC) includes a section giving advice regarding adverse drug reactions and their reporting, while the MHRA has resources for professionals about ADRs.

The risk of adverse events can be reduced by:

- only using a drug with a good indication and where the benefit outweighs the risk of side effects;
- using the lowest therapeutic dose for the shortest durations;
- checking if they have previous *allergies* or intolerances to medication, including additives or excipients or foods;
- confirming if they are taking any other medication, including those that they can buy, such as supplements or herbal medicines, as interactions could increase the risk of adverse drug reactions;
- considering if smaller doses are needed, due to age and hepatic or renal disease that may alter the metabolism or excretion of drugs.

Activity 5.7 asks you to think critically about adverse drug reactions in relation to the ibuprofen Madiba is taking.

Activity 5.7   Critical thinking

Madiba is now taking oral ibuprofen 400mg three times a day as required and has been taking it for several years. He states that on some of the days he takes ibuprofen he suffers from indigestion and gastro-intestinal discomfort.

- Do you think he is suffering from an adverse drug reaction caused by the ibuprofen tablets?
- If so, would you consider this to be a Type A or Type B reaction?
- What advice would you offer to Madiba to reduce the risk of an adverse drug reaction?

An outline answer is provided at the end of the chapter.

Reporting adverse drug reactions

Research into new or well-established drugs is unable to fully capture the ways in which drugs act or cause side effects. This makes it important to report adverse drug reactions, particularly new ones or in children. For example, miconazole was initially allowed for infants under four months until there was a reported case of near-choking, prompting a change to prescribing advice (BNF, JFC). An understanding of when and how to report adverse and allergic reactions is needed and can be found in the BNF (JFC) and on the MHRA website.

Activity 5.8 asks you to further explore adverse reactions, the pharmacology underpinning them and reporting mechanisms.

Activity 5.8   Reflection

We have discussed some basic pharmacology and outlined some areas of consideration for preventing adverse drug reactions. With your practice assessor, explore what sources of information you would access to support your drug choices, identify risks and report adverse drug reactions.

While no answer is given, there is a selection of recommended reading and useful websites at the end of the chapter.

Chapter summary

This chapter provided an overview some of the core pharmacological principles of pertinence to prescribing and medicines. Some of the processes involved are highly complex so

(Continued)

(Continued)

it is advisable to access other resources such as those listed at the end of the chapter, with the aim of ensuring you have a good grasp of any medicines you are accountable for administering or prescribing. A personal formulary (introduced in Chapter 7) can be an effective way to record and take notes about the medicines you are comfortable with pre-scribing, adding to this as your scope of practice expands.

Activities: suggested answers and discussion points

Answer to Activity 5.1 Critical thinking

For available forms of ibuprofen, dosing, advice, side effects, contra-indications, or concerns regarding his taking ibuprofen, the best sources of information are the BNF (JFC) or the elec-tronic Medicines Compendium (eMC) which holds the summary of product characteristics (SmPC) for the drug. This information would need to be taken in context of the person and their bio-psycho-social assessment as outlined in Chapter 3. Depending on its form and quantity, ibu-profen is a pharmacy (P), prescription-only medicine (POM), or available on the general sales list (GSL). It is important to note prescribing differences between preparations as not all of the listed indications/therapeutic uses in the BNF are prescribable by community practitioner prescribers. For ibuprofen, prescribing by community nurse prescribers is only for the indications and at the doses stated in the Nurse Prescribers' Formulary for Community Practitioners (NPFCP). These are the indications and doses that are not classified as POM. Some of the indications and doses in the ibuprofen entry in the BNF (JFC) are classified as POM and can only be legally prescribed by full formulary (non-medical/V300) prescribers. That is why the NPFCP has a maximum daily dose of 1.2g while in the BNF it is 2.4g, and why the indications vary.

Answer to Activity 5.2 Critical thinking

Examples of medicinal forms you may have thought of are found in Figure 5.1. The route of administration and medicinal form are important for several reasons including being patient-centred and ensuring you take account of the patient's beliefs and preferences.

- Some people will not be able to swallow tablets or capsules and will therefore need a liquid form of the medicine or to have it administered by another route.
- If the individual does not wish to take anything of porcine or bovine derivative (animal origin) for religious or other reasons, then you must be sensitive and know which medi-cines should be avoided. For example, many capsules would be unacceptable because of the gelatine and most of the low molecular weight heparins (LMWH) like enoxaparin sodium, dalteparin and tinzaparin are porcine derived.
- There may have been allergies/sensitivities to certain forms in the past. Many medicinal forms have soya or peanut oil as a constituent.

Answer to Activity 5.3 Critical thinking

Considering our case study of Madiba and the available forms of ibuprofen, there are a range of oral preparations (e.g. capsules, tablets, syrup, suspension) as well as topical gel. The oral formulations are rapidly absorbed from the gastro-intestinal tract. The active ingredient in the gel penetrates through the skin, making its way to the underlying soft tissues, joints and the synovial fluid. Absorption of the oral preparation is affected by such factors as: the preparation (e.g. whether enteric-coated), food or fluid in the stomach, gastric emptying, gastric pH, gastric motility. Absorption of the topical preparation is affected by temperature, blood flow, or skin conditions such as broken or damaged skin (where it is contra-indicated).

Answer to Activity 5.4 Critical thinking

Considering our case study of Madiba and the distribution of ibuprofen:

1. the SmPC (eMC, Medicines.org) states ibuprofen is extensively protein bound. In the interaction section, there are notable interactions with drugs such as warfarin (that is also highly protein bound), focused on the increased risk of bleeding events;

2. as an older person, it would be important to assess for signs of protein deficiency. For example, nutritional status, signs of oedema, co-morbidities of acute illness such as sepsis.

Answer to Activity 5.5 Critical thinking

An enzyme inducer catalyses (speeds up) the reaction between an enzyme (usually found in the liver) and its natural substrate or a drug, such as ibuprofen which is metabolised by cytochrome P450 CYP 2C9. As metabolism occurs at a faster rate, the substrate is broken down more quickly to produce a product, or the drug into its metabolite(s).

St John's wort is a herbal remedy available to purchase for the treatment of mild depression. It is known to be an enzyme inducer. In the BNF you will notice that St John's wort is predicted to decrease the exposure to many drugs, as it catalyses the reaction between the drug and its liver enzyme.

There are no interactions listed in Appendix 1 of the BNF between St John's wort and ibuprofen, although it is a general caution for use in the elderly. However, you may have read further that St John's wort does induce the enzyme CYP2C9 responsible for the metabolism of ibuprofen. This effect is not thought to significantly change the efficacy of ibuprofen and thus is not listed in the BNF.

Answer to Activity 5.6 Critical thinking

The excretion of ibuprofen is rapid and complete via the kidneys. As an older adult, Madiba is likely to have a degree of renal impairment and may not be keeping hydrated enough. There is a risk of papillary necrosis (kidney damage) from ibuprofen, especially in long-term use. Blood flow to the kidneys and co-morbidities such as heart failure or renal failure can affect renal excretion. An acute kidney injury will cause the excretion of ibuprofen to slow down or stop, with a risk of further damage. He should be advised to stop taking the ibuprofen (including any topical preparations) and ensure adequate fluid intake.

Answer to Activity 5.7 Critical thinking

Madiba could be experiencing an adverse drug reaction, and ibuprofen is advised for short-term use only. This would be an 'augmented' or Type A reaction. The advice would be to try the topical form or find an alternative medicine.

Further reading and useful websites

Knowing where to find reliable medicines information is essential for safe, person-centred prescribing, administration, advice, safety-netting and monitoring. There are excellent sources of information available to further your understanding of pharmacology, aid safe and effective prescribing and report adverse reactions. Some of the main information sources are listed, although it should be noted that another valuable source of information is pharmacists. They regularly provide advice about medicines to people receiving prescriptions as well as acting as expert advisors to prescribers.

The most important source of information is the British National Formulary (BNF), published by the Joint Formulary Committee (JFC) every six months. There is a separate BNF for Children (BNFc) and a Nurse Prescribers' Formulary (NPF). While the hard copy contains more information, they are also conveniently available online.

- The British National Formulary (BNF) (JFC). https://bnf.nice.org.uk
- The British National Formulary for Children (BNFc). https://bnfc.nice.org.uk
- Community Practitioner Nurse Prescribers' Formulary (NPF). https://bnf.nice.org.uk/nurse-prescribers-formulary/

It is also advisable to access manufacturers' SmPC and patient information leaflet (PIL) for additional information about specific products. The SmPC includes more detail about the pharmacology.

- Medicines Data sheets. Available from the electronic Medicines Compendium (eMC) (https://www.medicines.org.uk). These include both:
  - SmPC: for health professionals re. how to prescribe and use a medicine correctly. It is based on clinical trials and gives information about pharmacology, dose, use and side effects;
  - patient information leaflets: the leaflet included in the pack with a medicine; a summary of the SmPC written for patients.

Guidelines, local policies/formularies, alerts

National guidelines with respect to medicines and treatment choice are available from the National Institute of Health and Care Excellence (NICE) or the Scottish Intercollegiate Guidelines Network (SIGN). These provide a wide range of information sources and include the evidence base for recommended treatments.

- National Institute of Health and Care Excellence. www.NICE.org.uk
- Scottish Intercollegiate Guidelines Network. https://www.sign.ac.uk

NHS providers develop policies and formularies for prescribing. Formularies are often developed jointly between several care providers and detail preferred (or prohibited) products based on national guidelines (but can include local variations). You need to access your own organisation's prescribing policy. An example from a primary care provider is Derbyshire Medicines Management, Prescribing and Guidelines. This categorises medicines in five ways as to whether they 'approve' them for prescribing: GREEN (prescribable in primary care); AMBER (only prescribable in primary care after started by a consultant); RED (only prescribable in secondary care/by a consultant); GREY (exceptional circumstances only); DO NOT PRESCRIBE (DNP) (not recommended or commissioned).

- Derbyshire Medicines Management, Prescribing and Guidelines. http://www.derbyshiremedicinesmanagement.nhs.uk/medicines-management

Prescribers and practitioners must keep up to date with alerts from the MHRA as some alerts (Red) need acting upon within 24 hours, so can affect the medicines being prescribed or administered by you. These will normally be communicated via employers, but prescribers should sign up for these to be delivered automatically, as well as using the website as a source of pharmacological information. Another very useful resource is the Specialist Pharmacy Service (for all practitioners).

- Medicines and Healthcare Products Regulatory Agency (MHRA). https://www.gov.uk/government/organisations/medicines-and-healthcare-products-regulatory-agency
- Specialist Pharmacy Service. https://www.sps.nhs.uk/

Pharmacology textbooks and websites

Textbooks are a reliable source of core information for pharmacological principles. An example includes:

- Ashelford, S, Raynsford, J and Taylor, V (2019) *Pathophysiology and Pharmacology in Nursing* (2nd edn). London: Sage.
- https://www.vitalsource.com/en-uk/referral?term=9781526471376
- The pharmacology education project. https://www.pharmacologyeducation.org

People learn in diverse ways, so you may also find accessing a range of short video or e-learning tools to be beneficial to understanding pharmacology.

- Handwritten tutorials: a series of video tutorials, starting with pharmacokinetics. https://www.youtube.com/watch?v=8-Qtd6RhfVA
- Pharmacology tutorials. https://www.youtube.com/c/pharmacologytutorials/featured
- Study.com (a paid-for service, with a free trial). https://study.com/academy/topic/basics-of-pharmacology.html

Chapter 6　Teamwork, communication and public health

Introduction

Previous chapters discussed accountability for safe prescribing that includes sufficient understanding of consultation, evidence and pharmacology. As there are limits to our professional knowledge, safe and effective practice also requires good teamwork, communication and an awareness of these limitations. Clinical decision-making must also be aligned with the person's view of their health, or health beliefs, as well as the wider public health context. Equally the importance of choosing not to prescribe and consideration of non-pharmacological approaches such as social prescribing is essential to ensure evidence-based treatment options are used to support clinical decision-making. This chapter starts with an overview of the public health context of prescribing practice, briefly considers social prescribing and then discusses vaccination and antimicrobial stewardship as examples of health protection. The last sections examine communication and teamwork, with discussion of these in relation to remote consultations.

Public health practice

Scenario 6.1

You are a newly qualified nurse employed in the community setting. When you visit Mr James for the first time to undertake wound care you notice there is a distinct odour and other indications, such as darkly nicotine-stained fingers, to suggest he is likely a heavy smoker. As the visit progresses, you ask if he's aware of the harms of smoking and explain that it can cause poor wound healing. He says he does know and that he thought you were here for his dressing, not his smoking. A few days later, the district nurse tells you she has been to visit Mr James who said he doesn't want that *young cheeky nurse in his house again*.

While there is a balance between the care we need to perform, expectations of people in our care and professional requirements, public health should be embedded in all aspects of our practice (NMC 2018b, c; RPS, 2021a). Prescribing episodes can be seen as opportunities to promote health whether by proactively contributing to prevention strategies, facilitating self-care or improving access to services and reducing health inequalities. Prescribing practice involves aspects of public health such as medicines optimisation or de-prescribing, encouraging lifestyle alternatives or ensuring informed choice. The World Health Organization (WHO) (2018, p78) sets out some core values of health and healthcare, identifying that services should be *high quality, equitable, sustainable and universal.* Nurse and midwife prescribing is an effective, efficient and sustainable way to bring services closer to the people who need them, improving access and equity. In a similar way, NHS public health strategies aim for services that meet the 'triple aim' of better health and wellbeing for everyone (improved outcomes), better-quality health services (the person's experience of healthcare) and sustainable use of NHS resources (improved cost effectiveness) (DHSC, 2021b). V300, V150 and V100 prescribing has consistently evaluated as contributing positively to those aims, and holds potential to further contribute to the wider public health agenda.

The WHO have adopted Acheson's (1988) definition of public health as *the art and science of preventing disease, prolonging life and promoting health through the organised efforts of society.* The RCN (2016, p28) suggests public health shouldn't be seen as separate area of practice, as nurses *have the skills and are best placed to provide meaningful public health interventions* across all settings as part of person-centred care. They separate public health into the 'three Ps': promotion, prevention and protection (RCN, 2020b). Health inequalities can be seen to cut across a range of aspects (Acheson, 1998; Marmot et al., 2010, 2020; DoH, 2010; RCN, 2020b), so public health for prescribing is discussed in the context of three core purposes: health protection, health promotion (including prevention) and addressing inequalities. Activity 6.1 uses these three aspects of public health to prompt reflection on your practice as a future prescriber.

Activity 6.1 Reflection: your public health role

Three core public health functions for prescribers can be seen as health protection, health promotion and reducing inequalities by providing equitable services. Reflecting on a recent episode from practice, identify how you as a developing prescriber could meet one or more of these public health roles.

As this activity asks you to reflect on your practice, no answer is provided.

Activity 6.1 asked you to think about the public health aspects of your future prescribing. While it is recognised public health is everyone's responsibility some find the concept difficult to separate from clinical activities. Breaking it into the three roles of protection, promotion and inequalities can help better highlight where prescribing practice can contribute to the overarching aim of improving population health. These three themes are explored in more detail with a focus on medicines and prescribing.

Health protection

The clearest example of health protection is in strategies and the response to a global pandemic such as COVID-19. Health protection relates to effectively responding to outbreaks of infectious disease and other risks to population health (Griffith and Tengnah, 2017; RCN, 2021b), with activities including surveillance, screening, reporting (e.g. test and trace), monitoring and immunisation. Health protection legally entails reporting of 'notifiable diseases' (HPSC, 2021) aimed at preventing spread, facilitating early identification of outbreaks and supplying evidence for public health interventions such as immunisation.

Aspects of medicines management are pertinent to health protection, such as the 'cold chain' or correct handling of vaccines to ensure their efficacy during storage and transportation. Allen (2021) stresses the significance of effective medicines management for COVID-19 vaccines, stating it is essential to the success of the vaccination programme. Other examples of health protection include screening programmes that aim to detect and address health issues such as TB or cancer. For example, screening looks for findings that could indicate a specific cancer or pre-cancer before symptoms have developed, although this isn't suitable for all types (WHO, 2021a, b). In relation to prescribing, one of the most significant threats to public health is that of antimicrobial resistance (AMR) (WHO, 2020a, b).

Antimicrobial resistance

The WHO has identified AMR as one of the top ten global public health threats (WHO, 2020a, b). Public Health England (PHE, 2021) make a direct link between antibiotic prescribing and antibiotic resistance, stating that over-prescribing or incorrect use of antibiotics are key causes of resistance. There are published updates and indicators to raise awareness of antibiotic prescribing and this public health risk. For instance, in England the estimated number of antibiotic-resistant bacterial bloodstream infections increased by 32 per cent between 2015 and 2019, with an estimated 65,162 antibiotic-resistant severe infections in 2019 (nearly 200 per day) (PHE, 2020). While there has been an overall decline in antibiotic use since 2015, there is varying success in meeting national targets for this and resistance continues to grow (PHE, 2020). Guidelines, resources and tools have been made available to all prescribers, but a national survey showed that only 52 per cent of nurses correctly answered knowledge test questions about AMR compared with 80 per cent of doctors and 74 per cent of pharmacists (PHE, 2020), suggesting more needs to be done. Although the focus is primarily on systemically acting antibiotics, AMR should also be considered with topical antimicrobial products. For example, in leg ulcer treatment the BNF (JFC) warns that topical antibacterials should normally be avoided and that treatment of bacterial colonisation (as opposed to infection) is generally inappropriate. NICE (2016a) also advises to limit the choice of topical antibacterials to those that are not used systemically.

Antimicrobial stewardship

Antimicrobial stewardship is a system-wide approach to promote and monitor the use of antimicrobials to preserve their future effectiveness (RPS, 2021a). Courtenay and Chater (2021) mention that nurses are increasingly involved in antibiotic prescribing, such as for wound care, respiratory or urinary tract infections, all of which have been shown to develop bacterial resistance to antibiotics. This reinforces the need to gain competence in this area of prescribing practice – for example, recognising symptoms when determining a working diagnosis of viral or bacterial infection. Nurses are in a good position to provide advice and explain judicious use of antibiotics which can be aided by a competency framework (Courtenay and Chater, 2021). Specific antimicrobial prescribing competencies should be used alongside the prescribing competency framework (PHE, 2013; NHS Scotland, 2014; NICE, 2019b). The CFAP (RPS, 2021a) explicitly acknowledges antimicrobial resistance and the roles of infection prevention, control and antimicrobial stewardship measures. An outline of some of the guidance, resources and learning aids can be found in the Further reading section of this chapter. Activity 6.2 asks you to self-assess your current knowledge and competence around antimicrobial stewardship

---

Activity 6.2   Reflection – Antimicrobial stewardship competencies

AMS is an important aspect of practice that you have likely already encountered or received some training for. Access a competency framework for AMS (found in Further reading at the end of the chapter) and self-assess your learning needs as a future prescriber.

Activity 6.2 asked you to self-assess your professional development needs in relation to AMS, so no answer is provided. You may wish to discuss your self-assessment with your practice assessor. Resistance by bacterial organisms is an important global health risk that prescribing professionals have a responsibility to understand and improve. We have discussed various aspects of health protection including AMS and will now look at health promotion and prevention.

Health promotion

An early psychological theory held that people either have an internal or external locus of control (Rotter, 1954). While this is a continuum, at the extreme ends a person with a strong external locus of control believes events are outside of their influence and are most likely to say *just tell me what do – it's up to you, you are the expert.* Someone at the other extreme may pay no attention whatsoever to clinical advice, as their strong internal locus of control means they believe to be in charge of their destiny. People at this end may refuse or demand inappropriate treatments. While people vary over time and differ individually, attitudes towards public health and health services are changing as people become less likely to see themselves as passive recipients of care. They may still seek advice and value expertise, but the role of professionals is moving towards collaboration with people and communities to improve health and wellbeing. Among other things, this may include strengthening self-efficacy (such as through motivational interviewing), building resilience, promoting healthy lifestyles, providing advice to facilitate self-care and ensuring accessibility of services (Dickson and Peelo-Kilroe, 2021). As introduced in Chapter 3, the consultation should start with rapport and attempting to gather the person's view of their health issue and priorities. This lends itself to opportunities for discussions focused on what matters most to the person in your care, offering the possibility of promoting health, or uncovering views on lifestyle change as one possible solution.

Health promotion can be seen to include aspects of behaviour change and prevention. For example, many long-term health conditions and some cancers have been linked to dietary and other lifestyle factors that can respond to changes in behaviour. This has resulted in behaviour change strategies being embedded in a range of national guidance, with NICE (2021b) linking it to at least 30 of their 'products'. For example, NICE (2017b) includes it in guidance on changing risk-related behaviours for antimicrobial stewardship and in their quality standard aimed at preventing premature mortality in minority ethnic groups (NICE, 2018b). While lifestyle and other non-medical interventions can't be recommended to everyone, there is a growing need to consider these as part of shared decision-making as they could have a significant effect. Depending at what stage they occur, it can be useful to think of health promotion and prevention as primary, secondary and tertiary. Primary prevention tends to be less expensive overall and more effective in lowering morbidity and mortality (WHO, 2020c). Some examples of each of the three levels are found in Table 6.1.

Primary prevention	Secondary prevention	Tertiary prevention
Immunisation	Cervical screening	Rehabilitation
Regular exercise	Breast or testicular self-examination	Self-care of a long-term condition
Healthy diet		

Table 6.1 Primary, secondary and tertiary prevention

Primary prevention could involve encouraging someone to change diet and lifestyle to prevent Type 2 diabetes linked to obesity. While lifestyle changes can prevent its development, they have also been found to repair some existing damage so that medicines are not required. People are said to have reversed their diabetes when they have been diagnosed with Type 2 but are able to get their blood glucose levels back to normal levels without taking diabetes medication (Diabetes UK, 2019). This normally involves loss of body weight through exercise and dietary changes (or bariatric surgery).

Social prescribing

In addition to healthy lifestyle changes, the bio-psycho-social model of health reminds us that there are other influences on a person's health and an interconnectivity between these aspects. For instance, social isolation has been recognised as contributing towards adverse quality of life outcomes, including poor physical and mental health (Luo *et al.*, 2012), hypertension (Hawkley *et al.*, 2010), heart disease (Xia and Li, 2018), depression, functional decline (Perissinoto *et al.*, 2012) and premature mortality (Day *et al.*, 2020). Assessing for these wider contributors to health and considering 'social prescribing' provides more options than a purely biological or medical model and can be a substitute for the prescription of drugs or medical intervention. NHS England (2019) identifies social prescribing as a strategy to involve people in their care, alongside shared decision-making, personalised care, etc., where people can be referred to various local, non-clinical services. Through recognising a multitude of ways in which people's health is determined, the aim is to take a more holistic approach to address concerns and support individuals in taking greater control of their own health (The King's Fund, 2017). Social prescribing schemes include activities such as volunteering, arts activities, group learning, gardening, befriending, cookery, healthy eating advice and sports (The King's Fund, 2017). Although it is preferable to be able to refer to such a scheme, evidence suggests that some activities on their own such as gardens and the arts are beneficial to the quality of life for older people or those with ill-health (While, 2020). A review by the WHO (Fancourt and Finn, 2019, p21) showed how *arts engagement can enhance multidimensional subjective well-being* and even just listening to music improves sleep, helps stroke recovery and can have an impact on dementia (While, 2020).

Equity and equality

Prescribing practice might not at first seem linked to health inequalities, but these can also be associated with access to healthcare. The expansion of prescribing by a wider range of practitioners has enabled care closer to home and quicker access to prescriptions. Addressing health inequalities includes targeting vulnerable populations, addressing inequity of service provision and promoting human rights where appropriate. Clinical guidelines are one way in which people should receive equitable, standardised care, although this is more difficult when services such as operations, products or medicines are not available between one area and another, often referred to as the 'postcode lottery'. As a prescriber, this may cause an ethical dilemma as illustrated by Activity 6.3.

Activity 6.3   Critical thinking: justice and equity

You are a community nurse prescriber (V150) and your geographical area of practice crosses a defined boundary. Velcro wrap compression is available to manage venous leg ulcers in place of four-layer compression bandaging in one area but not the other due to cost implications. Someone in the area where it isn't available is adamant you should prescribe that item for them. Critically consider with your practice assessor what might be done in this situation, and what it means for your duty of care.

No answer is provided for this activity.

Prescribing also needs to be individualised and has implications for human rights. For instance, there is a duty to ensure people are informed of products or their excipients that may have ingredients that impact on their philosophical, cultural or religious beliefs. There are quite a number of medicines that are bovine (beef) or porcine (pork) derived (or contain derivatives), including many vaccines. Taylor (2021) found it wasn't always possible to provide definitive information about whether animal products and alcohol are involved in the manufacturing processes of medicines, although it can be seen as part of a prescriber's duty of care to include questions about dietary restrictions or personal preferences. Taylor (2021, p6) suggests this should be done sensitively *because it may raise concerns people have not previously considered*. However, ethically we shouldn't withhold information, particularly when it is requested and this may involve contacting companies directly to gather data and being able to support individuals with their choices. We also have a professional duty to challenge false information while respecting people's preferences. Activity 6.4 invites you to consider information-giving further.

Activity 6.4   Critical thinking: vegan medicines

You are a new prescriber reviewing Miss J's medicines. She informs you she has recently become vegan for philosophical reasons and wants to know if any of her medicines contain or are made with animal or dairy products. Where would you look for that information in the first instance? How would you approach the situation if it transpired one of her required medicines was not vegan and there was no close alternative?

There is no answer provided for this activity, but you are encouraged to discuss this with your practice assessor or clinical pharmacist.

In Activity 6.4 we considered how to approach a situation where it can be difficult to find information, or know what alternatives there are. Good communication in such instances is crucial, along with the recognition of knowledge limits and when to seek the support of others. The next section expands on this theme of teamwork and communication as a way to improve prescribing practice, health outcomes and the person's experience of care.

Teamwork and communication

As a prescriber you will be acting independently and sometimes in isolation, but you are likely to be part of a team. Definitions of teams normally identify a group of people with shared aims, goals or tasks (Lynas, 2013). Health practitioners mainly work in a multi-disciplinary way, though not necessarily collaboratively (Chamberlain-Salaun *et al.*, 2013), but good teamworking has been found to result in better experiences for staff and the people in their care (Baird *et al.*, 2020). It has been noted that working as a team in a supportive environment lessens stress and has a positive influence on care. West (2021) outlines strategies for effective teamworking while under pressure during challenging times such as the COVID crisis – for example, focusing on competencies, supporting each other (showing compassion), clarifying team purpose, objectives and roles.

Groups simply working together can make teamwork appear to be ineffectual, when it is more likely they are not working in a 'real' team – that is, working closely, to shared aims and meeting regularly to review performance and objectives (West and Lyubovnikova, 2012). Øvretveit (1997) defines this type of arrangement as a 'network association', where professionals are loosely connected through working for the same client group. Due to how health services are funded, there can be competition between teams or even within multi-disciplinary teams where funding streams prompt different objectives. Health policies can also display recognition of the value of integration, with a shift towards primary care networks, community-based services and outpatient or specialist services that strengthen the benefits of professionals working collaboratively (Ham *et al.*, 2017; Charles, 2021; DHSC, 2021c). As a prescriber in this context, multi-disciplinary teams can be a good source of support for delivering best practice. An understanding of roles and responsibilities is essential within teams, but there also needs to be a focus on effective communication between team members (Baird *et al.*, 2020). Prescribing entails additional accountability but risks can be lessened and clinical outcomes improved through good teamwork and communication. Activity 6.5 uses the example of Mrs Smith to consider the wider team involved in people's care.

Activity 6.5 Critical thinking: multi-disciplinary teams

Mrs Smith is living with her daughter following the death of her husband from cancer. Her daughter contacted the GP to let them know her mum hasn't been eating well, is more forgetful, seems to be low in mood and is worried because the podiatrist hasn't been back to see her poorly toe. Thinking about services that may have been involved previously or for her own ongoing health issues, consider who in the wider multi-disciplinary team might contribute to her care. Who could be involved in prescribing for her health issues? How would you know what else has been prescribed or other advice that was provided?

Some suggestions are made at the end of the chapter.

Activity 6.5 asked you to critically consider the team involved with the care of Mrs Smith as an example of how the wider multi-disciplinary team can impact on your prescribing. When teams are working collaboratively and communicating effectively they can be of great benefit and provide support for your prescribing practice. Conversely, Lencioni (2002) identifies dysfunctions of a team that can cause stress and poor outcomes, including an absence of trust, fear of conflict, lack of commitment, avoidance of accountability and inattention to results (or outcomes). Seeking advice for an area of prescribing would be more challenging without a colleague or supervisor whose judgement you trusted, or if they lacked commitment and avoided accountability. Fear of conflict is much noted in the health service; part 9 of the Code attends to this, stating nurses must *provide honest, accurate and constructive feedback to colleagues* and *deal with differences of professional opinion* (NMC, 2018a, p10). Differences or variety in the wider multi-disciplinary team adds benefit when there is good communication and respect for each other's roles, creating efficiency and providing access to a depth and breadth of professional expertise.

We have looked at how the nature of the team you work within can impact on care provision. As a prescriber, you will benefit from and may be reliant on others to assure safe and effective prescribing practice. Activity 6.6 asks you to reflect on your practice situation in relation to support and advice.

Activity 6.6   Reflection: advice

As part of professionalism, prescribers are expected to continue developing competence and expand their scope of practice (as appropriate). Thinking about your current or future practice area, who might you approach for support? What are the attributes you would like to see in someone you would ask for advice? Now, turn this around and consider your own approach to practice. Are you someone whom others seek advice from? What aspects of your knowledge, skills or other attributes might you want to develop to become a team member whom others can rely on for sound advice?

There is no answer provided for this activity but you may wish to discuss with your practice assessor. Chapter 8 considers continuing professional development further.

Activity 6.6 asked you to identify qualities that would be beneficial in prescribers and the people they work with to help assure safe and effective prescribing. One of the themes that occurs regularly in relation to teamwork, as well as with consultation skills and behaviour change techniques, is that of communication. Unsurprisingly, communication is cited by many as key to a well-functioning team (Barr and Dowding, 2012; West and Lyubovnikova, 2013). It is also recognised as protective against errors, as, for example, research into medication errors shows that they can occur anywhere in the process due to poor or miscommunication (Elliot *et al.*, 2018). Examples of transition errors include a lack of communication about discharge prescriptions or medicines stopped during hospital admission (Keers *et al.*, 2015). It is worth being mindful of the likelihood of other prescribers prior to prescribing and asking the key questions such as whether there are any other involved professionals (RPS, 2021a). Where care is provided by a variety of teams and services, documentation is a vital form of communication, as well as being a legal requirement. It is recommended you find out about access to multi-disciplinary or multi-agency prescribing meetings or networking opportunities (this can also form part of your CPD). By being familiar with the RPS Framework (2021a) you will understand that all professionals in the UK adhere to this and therefore the quality of prescribing should be consistent across the board.

We have discussed teams, teamwork and communication; the next section explores types of communication using remote prescribing as an example where there are known barriers.

Types of communication and remote consultation

Effective communication is fundamental to being able to fulfil a duty of care through listening, observation, being attentive to cues when assessing, followed by being clear and precise with advice or treatment plans, and completing accurate contemporaneous documentation. Communication is an important skill used in daily practice with colleagues and the people in your care with many benefits for both. For practitioners, effective communication can improve confidence, job satisfaction and team cohesion as well as reducing stress. For the people in our care, it can reduce errors, enhance their experiences of care, reduce complaints, improve informed choice, reduce distress and aid concordance (McDonald, 2016). In contrast, poor communication is thought to cost the NHS over £1 billion per year; compromises adherence to medication regimes; results in repeat visits; and can lead to litigation (McDonald, 2016).

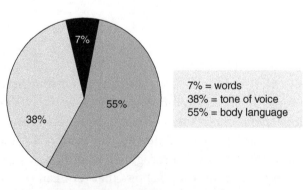

Figure 6.1 Non-verbal communication (Mehrabian, 1972)

Communication is normally seen as non-verbal, verbal or oral and written. While good listening skills are fundamental to success, the importance of non-verbal communication, including visual cues and tone, is notable. This is particularly true when there is discordance between what people are saying and their 'body language', as shown in Figure 6.1.

Non-verbal communication

Ali (2017) outlines the features of non-verbal communication, including eye contact, facial expressions, body or hand movements such as fidgeting, tremor/shaking, guarding and posture. These can change the meaning and can provide important cues to how someone is feeling. For example, someone may say they are not in pain, but their body language suggests otherwise. Body language also shows that you are actively listening. For example, it is important to avoid poor posture, be positive by smiling and making eye contact as appropriate, avoid fidgeting or looking your phone or watch and when you do need to leave, express this clearly. At times we can misinterpret non-verbal cues such as assuming someone is angry when they are upset or nervous. In this instance, open questions such as asking how they are can be helpful (Ali, 2017).

Verbal communication

As per Figure 6.1, verbal communication includes both the content of the message and how it's delivered. Because we use verbal communication so extensively, we may assume no further development is required. However, it is important to be aware of barriers and self-aware of ways to continue to improve. For example, with extensive documentation and assessment templates available there is a risk of not attending to the important job of active listening. This can include refraining from expressing your assumptions or reaching conclusions prematurely, showing a genuine interest in the person you are listening to and being empathic (NHS England and NHS Improvement, 2017). It is summed up by remembering that hearing is not listening. Paraphrasing or summarising in a consultation can demonstrate you have been listening, understood the intended meaning, while allowing the person to provide further clarification or information as needed.

Written communication

As professionals we are aware of the vital importance of clear, concise and precise documentation due to legal and professional requirements (NMC, 2018a; RPS, 2021a). It is not only pertinent for when things go wrong, but also a good way to communicate with others who may be involved in the person's care. From a team or colleague perspective, it is helpful to remember that written messages such as emails can have unintended meanings or more of an impact than if they were communicated verbally.

Remote consultation for prescribing

Prior to the COVID-19 pandemic, the work of most healthcare practitioners would primarily have been face to face. The exception to this is those working in NHS 111, whose consultations are undertaken by telephone. While this clearly requires a different approach and the development of skills to compensate for missing information, it is important to also note that of the 60,000–80,000 telephone contacts per day, approximately 85 per cent of these are onward-referred to other services (NHS England, 2021b). This reminds that for this service, and others, there are limitations to what can be achieved remotely. However, through improved telephone techniques, and additional technical solutions such as remote video, etc., the wider health service is adapting to remote consultation and finding some advantages.

For prescribing, there remain risks as outlined by joint agreed professional/NMC (2019b) high-level guidance for remote consultation. The RCN provides a good overview of pointers to keep in mind when undertaking a remote consultation for prescribing, and this is referenced in the Further reading section. A summary of advice follows the RAPID assessment as outlined in Chapter 3, with some of these additional points:

- ensuring you identify who you are speaking to – it may be a family member who decides to call on the person's behalf, and there may be consent implications, such as parental rights, or mental capacity issues;
- eliciting information about the presenting complaint and its history is likely to be the same, although you will have to listen out for any additional cues;
- the physical examination will differ, with the RCN (2020a) denoting this activity as 'indirect'. This refers to attaining the information by asking the patient to describe their signs and symptoms, and following up with specific questions. For example, if they mention a sore area on their lower leg, you would need to follow up with questions about warmth, location, if it's reddened, broken skin, leakage, etc. Questions may also include home readings and, where possible, the use of video conferencing can be helpful. Listening for breathing, tone of voice and background noise can also help, particularly in the absence of other cues;
- the diagnosis may need to be a provisional or working diagnosis, but can still determine actions. For example, you may conclude the person needs to be seen/ be referred or that there are sufficient signs of a wound infection, for example, for which antibiotics are warranted, but this is in the absence of a wound swab;
- treatment and safety-netting must be particularly clear and it needs to be established that the person understands the actions to take (worsening advice);
- prescriptions, documentation and follow-up needs to be clear.

Although remote prescribing may not be appropriate for your area of practice, it has shown that prescriptions can be obtained in alternative ways if necessary. McKenna (2020) noted an increase of 8.5 million prescribed items (9.3 per cent) in March 2020 and additional costs of £118 million (17.6 per cent) compared to March 2019, with some items such as paracetamol or salbutamol inhalers showing significant increases. It is likely there will be a mix of face-to-face and remote consultations as people appreciate the convenience of not having to travel to seek health services. As a prescriber, it is advisable to hone communication skills and prepare for questions and possible uncertainty or unrealistic expectations that remote consultations for prescribing can prompt.

Chapter summary

This chapter explored public health aspects of prescribing, and features of good teamwork and communication. The person's perspective and identifying when to offer non-pharmacological solutions were discussed. The last sections examined concepts of teams and communication with some discussion of remote consultations. The next chapter applies the principles discussed throughout the preceding chapters to a range of prescribing scenarios.

Activities: suggested answers and discussion points

Answer to Activity 6.5 Critical thinking: multi-disciplinary teams

Mrs Smith is likely to have a wide number of practitioners involved in her care, although they can only be loosely referred to as a team. For instance, while her husband was alive, she is likely to have had support from the Macmillan and district nursing teams and, depending on the situation, this support sometimes continues to help deal with bereavement and grief. Relatedly, she will be followed by her GP, and may be on anti-depressants along with other medications for a variety of medical conditions. Depending on her clinical history, she may also be prescribed for by a consultant or other specialist, such as for dementia care. Depending on circumstances, she may have been supported by adult social care, dementia care or clinical, such as a leg ulcer club. While most prescriptions should be noted on her GP care record, it is possible for some of these to be missed – for example, products issued from stock in a leg ulcer clinic, or antibiotics supplied by a podiatrist as they are able to supply antibiotics for foot conditions without the need for a prescription.

Further reading and useful websites

We explored the concept of antimicrobial resistance. There are several learning tools and resources available with some of the recommended reading provided.

Antimicrobial resistance (AMR). https://www.gov.uk/health-and-social-care/antimicrobial-resistance

Future Learn: antimicrobial and antibiotic resistance courses. https://www.futurelearn.com/subjects/healthcare-medicine-courses/antimicrobial-and-antibiotic-resistance

Future Learn: evolving stewardship – roles in the antimicrobial management team. https://www.futurelearn.com/info/courses/antimicrobial-stewardship/0/steps/7519

NICE guidance (collection). Antimicrobial stewardship https://www.nice.org.uk/guidance/conditions-and-diseases/infections/antimicrobial-stewardship

National Institute for Health and Care Excellence (NICE) (2020e) *Leg Ulcer Infection: Antimicrobial Prescribing*. NICE guideline [NG152]. https://www.nice.org.uk/guidance/ng152

Health Education (collection). England Antimicrobial resistance; includes an e-learning package. https://www.hee.nhs.uk/our-work/antimicrobial-resistance

World Health Organization (WHO) (2017) *WHO publishes list of bacteria for which new antibiotics are urgently needed*. https://www.who.int/news/item/27-02-2017-who-publishes-list-of-bacteria-for-which-new-antibiotics-are-urgently-needed

https://www.england.nhs.uk/publication/social-prescribing-link-workers/

Remote prescribing

RCN (2020) *Prescribing safely under COVID-19.*

https://www.rcn.org.uk/clinical-topics/medicines-management/covid-19-remote-prescribing

Chapter 7

The Nurse Prescribers' Formulary

Chapter aims

After reading this chapter, you will be able to:

- apply consultation frameworks and evidence-informed practice to prescribing;
- identify influences on person-centred clinical decision-making;
- outline how to promote safe and effective treatment, advice-giving, safety-netting, follow-up and monitoring.

Introduction

Scenario

You have recently qualified as a registered nurse and started working with a small district nursing team in a rural area. As a qualified specialist practitioner (SPQ–DN) the team leader is a community formulary (V100) prescriber. However, she is quite busy so visits have had to be delayed due to products such as catheters and dressings needing to be prescribed. Although you would like to eventually prescribe from the full BNF, you can see the benefits of prescribing the range of products from the Nurse Prescribers' Formulary and are interested in developing competence for these.

As outlined in the opening chapter, nurses and midwives are expected to be 'prescribing ready' at the point of registration, though need to undertake a prescribing course and develop their competence to safely expand their scope of practice. While standards are constantly evolving, from 1994 community formulary (V100/V150) prescribing was integral to the District Nurse Specialist Practice Qualification (SPQ). To illustrate the transition from qualified nurse to prescriber, this chapter starts with a brief overview of the Nurse Prescribers' Formulary for Community Practitioners (NPF) before applying core prescribing principles to a practice example.

In previous chapters, we have examined wide-ranging influences on clinical decision-making, including for prescribing. In this chapter, clinical scenarios are used to illustrate a systematic approach to prescribing, which can be adapted to a range of situations and products. While examples are drawn from the NPF, key points of consideration can be applied to wider practice situations. As encounters with people in your care always entail a clinical decision, it is important to be aware of the options including taking no action, providing advice, de-prescribing or issuing a prescription within your current qualification and scope of practice. This chapter explores influences on your clinical decision-making, including legal, ethical and professional considerations, person-centred consultation, pharmacology and evidence-informed practice.

A number of the RPS (2021a) prescribing competencies are addressed, including the stages of assessment and decision-making as illustrated by the RAPID-CASE model detailed in Chapter 3. This model is used to frame the discussion of the scenarios, with aspects of governance referred to where appropriate. Although the examples use products from the Nurse Prescribers' Formulary, they are available for all prescribers and concern commonly encountered ailments. One detailed example is provided as a template for other areas of prescribing that you may encounter. This is aided by the continuing professional development tool, the *personal formulary* discussed later in this chapter. As a prescriber it is important to identify what can help reassure you that your prescriptions are safe, appropriate and effective. Using a consistent approach and recording this in a personal formulary is an effective way to document and help assure your preparedness for expanding your scope of prescribing practice.

Nurse Prescribers' Formulary for Community Practitioners (NICE, NPAG)

An independent prescriber is defined by the RPS (2021a, p21) as a *prescribing healthcare professional who is responsible and accountable for the assessment of patients with undiagnosed or diagnosed conditions and for decisions about the clinical management required, including prescribing.* They go on to define the two distinct forms of 'non-medical' prescribers as independent prescribers and community practitioner nurse prescribers (CPNPs). The NPF provides a list of preparations legally approved for prescribing by CPNPs, but in some cases only for specified indications. For example, aspirin can be prescribed for mild to moderate pain or pyrexia, but not at doses or for indications linked to cardiovascular health. The NPF is overseen by the Nurse Prescribers' Advisory Group who advises UK health ministers on the list of preparations (NICE, NPAG). The basic list only contains about 45 products, but there are various sub-groups such as types of emollients and nearly 600 pages in the Drug Tariffs (across the four countries) detailing products like dressings, appliances and chemical reagents. Despite this wide array of products, there are relatively few items in the NPF that work systemically. Whether prescribing products that act locally or medicines with a systemic effect, a thorough approach to prescribing is required.

In previous chapters we have looked at aspects of prescribing for some of the products in the NPF, including head lice (for making a diagnosis), emollients (in relation to evidence-based practice), or analgesia (ibuprofen – pharmacology). For this chapter, the main example will be laxatives, while other products from the NPF such as emollients, nicotine replacement therapy, wound care and appliances will be briefly outlined. Like the BNF, the NPF (NICE, NPAG) includes general advice and treatment summaries, but these are very basic so additional information should always be sought. Activity 7.1 asks you to reflect on practice from the perspective of a prescriber.

Activity 7.1   Reflection

Consider a recent example from your practice and the questions below. Asking these should enable you to reflect on when prescribing would be beneficial and whether it is a suitable area to start your prescribing.

- What was the presenting problem?
- Were you able to identify key issues and confirm a diagnosis?

(Continued)

(Continued)

- If the treatment decision involved prescribing, were you comfortable in knowing what was needed?
- Were there any aspects that needed further information or study before you would be able to prescribe in this situation?

As this activity is based on your own reflection there is no sample answer provided at the end of the chapter. You may wish to discuss this activity with a practice colleague.

Keep your reflection on practice from Activity 7.1 in mind when reading through the case study presented below and across the range of topics. As a reminder, Figure 1.1 in Chapter 1 illustrates governance forming the foundation of prescribing practice. For any practice scenario, we need to start by considering these issues followed by the steps to decision-making structured by the RAPID-CASE model.

Scenario: laxatives (adults)

Scenario 7.2   The de Silva family – Mr Mohammed (Mo) de Silva

You are a community staff nurse visiting Mrs Smith who lives with her daughter and the rest of the de Silva family. During the visit, Mr de Silva (Mo) asks to speak to you in private. He seems agitated and reluctant to speak. After several attempts, he finally tells you that he thinks he might be constipated because he hasn't gone to the toilet in several days and would like some advice.

Governance

Starting with governance issues, the following questions would need to be considered before proceeding with a consultation.

- Do you owe him a duty of care?
- Are you the right person to undertake this consultation? Is this within your scope of practice?
- Is this the right place? Should he be referred?
- Does he have the mental capacity to consent?

Although Mo isn't formally on your 'caseload', people can self-refer to community nursing services and as he has asked you for advice, some type of decision would need to be made and documented. Ethical, legal and professional principles would indicate you owe a duty of care, even if this is fulfilled by onward referral. While it is important to undertake consultation in the appropriate setting (RPS, 2021a), there may be little choice for individuals in receipt of community nursing services who primarily or exclusively receive care in their own home. In this instance, Mo declines to visit the general practitioner (GP) and consents to an assessment for his presenting complaint of possible constipation.

The consultation

In this scenario you consider assessing someone with constipation to be within your scope of practice and you agree to undertake the consultation with Mo. If this were a child, or outside of your scope for another reason, it would be important to explain this, refer and document any advice provided. The following questions would need to be considered for the consultation.

- Can privacy and dignity be maintained?
- Do you have access to his medical notes/records?
- Are you up to date with assessing for constipation?
- Do you have access to information or support available if issues occur that you are uncomfortable with?

As detailed in Chapter 3, a structured approach to the assessment should be taken, particularly when the person you are assessing is unknown to you, or a new problem has arisen. Using the RAPID-CASE consultation model (Figure 7.1), an overview of an example structured assessment is provided.

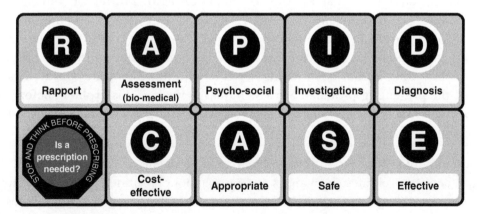

Figure 7.1 RAPID-CASE consultation model for prescribing

Rapport/initial stages

In this scenario, introductions would have been made on previous visits or when assistance was requested, although clarification of your role, the possible need for referral and time limits should be indicated. Confirming identification helps check records and is needed for documentation. While mental capacity is assumed, basic questions around his understanding of the situation and the need for an assessment can help confirm this (NICE, 2018a). Consent should be obtained and documented alongside appropriate clinical details or any prescribed treatment. Having gained consent and assessed mental capacity, you can explore Mo's view of the health issue using open questions and using the ICE (ideas, concerns and expectations) acronym.

Mo reports he has been feeling generally low and hasn't been leaving the house much. Because of some back pain and the family situation he hasn't been as physically active as usual, so thinks this may be why he's having trouble going to the toilet (ideas). He says his main concern is that it will get worse and he will have to go into hospital (concerns) and he would like it to be treated as soon as possible (expectations).

Assessment of biomedical

Now that you have established Mo's perception of the main problem the assessment should move on to a mix of focused questions to gather specific information along with continued use of open questions as appropriate. You will want to establish basic information such as relevant medical history, allergies and medication history, including any purchased (over the counter) or herbal preparations, before further exploration of the presenting complaint. You will also want to know whether he has had this problem before in the past and, if so, what helped to resolve it.

On taking Mo's medical and medication history, he says he has cut down on his smoking but is not very active due to back pain from an old sports injury. He is taking some paracetamol for this along with codeine as prescribed by his GP. You check his understanding of paracetamol dose limits as per BNF (JFC, NICE), whether he is taking any other products that contain paracetamol, as well as reviewing adherence to and effectiveness of his prescribed analgesia. Assessment should include duration, such as how long he has been taking codeine, and its effectiveness, as well as history of the presenting problem. Mo says he has never had this problem before, and it is also the first time he has had to take medicine stronger than paracetamol for his back pain.

Information of pertinence to this problem includes dietary habits and changes, fluid intake, activity level, lifestyle changes and normal bowel routine. Although diagnostic criteria for constipation include bowel movements being fewer than three times per week, it is often defined as less frequently than the person's normal pattern (NICE CKS, 2020a). In addition to frequency, the type or consistency of bowel movements help with diagnosis so you would need to assess this preferably using a recognised tool such as the Bristol stool chart (NICE CKS, 2020a) to aid documentation. You would also check for associated symptoms such as loss of appetite, nausea, vomiting, confusion, overflow diarrhoea, urinary retention or abdominal pain, discomfort, bloating or distension (RCN, 2019b; NICE CKS, 2020a).

Psycho-social and context

Further information of pertinence can be gained through a more conversational approach to identify other influences on the presenting problem(s). Mo reports no medical issues in his family history. He says he has felt more stressed since being out of work, at home with the three children all the time and his mother-in-law recently moving into the family home. Depression or anxiety requires assessment and can have an impact on physical wellbeing, including perception of pain, and is a risk factor for constipation (NICE CKS, 2020a). The person's main concern can be their mental health, with the physical ailment being secondary, so it is important to explore this within the limits of your scope of practice. Physical activity is known to improve mild depression, so advice may be indicated. However, in this scenario guidance would need to take into account other problems such as old injuries and back pain, so referral back to the GP or a team approach is most appropriate. The assessment in this instance suggests Mo may have mild depression, but is not at current risk, so you recommend he discuss this with his GP and gain his agreement to continue discussing his presenting problem of possible constipation.

Investigations/clinical examination(s)

From what you have gathered through history-taking leads you to identify a working diagnosis of constipation secondary to opioid use and reduced physical activity. It is always important to consider and rule out other causes (differential diagnoses), either through investigations, examination, further enquiry or by trying a particular treatment. Before moving on to physical examination, Activity 7.2 asks you to identify some red and amber flag symptoms, or potential causes for referral.

Activity 7.2   Decision-making: identifying red and amber flag symptoms

Constipation may be an underlying symptom of other issues or there can be associated signs that require further investigation. Identify what causes for concern could prompt urgent referral (red flags) in an adult. Consider if there are additional concerns for children – noted as red or amber in the constipation in children guidance (NICE CKS, 2020b).

An answer to Activity 7.2 is provided at the end of the chapter.

Activity 7.2 asked you to identify some situations where you may need to stop and consider urgent or non-urgent referral. Before outlining physical examination to aid diagnosis, a brief overview of the physiology is provided. Knowledge of underlying anatomy, physiology and pathophysiology is required in order to more fully understand treatment options. This applies to your future prescribing, although it is acknowledged that for some medicines or products, the precise mechanism of action is poorly understood.

Anatomy, physiology and pathophysiology of constipation

It is helpful for understanding causes of constipation and best treatment options to know how the large bowel functions, what may cause problems and how these can be resolved. As per Figure 7.2, the large bowel starts with the caecum, extends upwards via the ascending colon, across the transverse colon to the descending colon, past the sigmoid flexure, to the rectum, where the stool exits the body through the anus. Partially digested food materials (chyme) pass from the small intestine into the caecum via the ileo-caecal valve, where it is stored until moving into the ascending colon. The appendix which has no known function is at the blind-ending pouch end of the caecum.

Structure

As per Figure 7.3, the intestinal wall broadly has the same structure as other parts of the GI tract, although the mucosa has a smooth absorptive surface rather than villi (like the small intestine). The large intestine has a puckered appearance because the three long, smooth muscle bands known as the taeniae coli aren't as long as the colon itself. The taenia coli become a continuous muscular layer in the rectum.

Functions of the bowel

The three main functions of the large intestine are absorption of water and electrolytes, formation and transit of faeces, and chemical digestion by gut microbes.

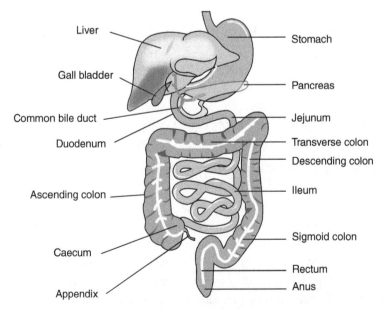

Figure 7.2   Organs of the GI tract (Ashelford *et al.*, 2019)

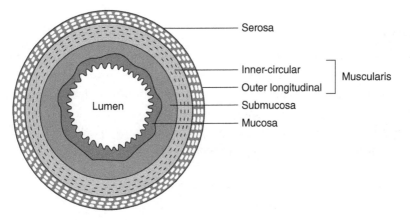

Figure 7.3 Layers of the wall of the GI tract (Ashelford *et al.*, 2019)

Most fluid absorption and food digestion has already occurred before its journey through the colon. Only a portion of the food residue and water that enters the caecum each day will eventually be eliminated, with most of the water and debris being absorbed. Solids are a mix of bacteria, undigested food fibre (cellulose), epithelial cells, small amounts of fats, proteins and the breakdown products from red blood cells (which cause its mainly brown colour). Mucous is secreted to maintain colonic pH and lubricate the faeces so they can pass through more easily. Movement through the intestine is relatively slow with the journey from eating to eliminating 70 per cent of a meal estimated at about three days (Nigam *et al.*, 2019), although this will vary. Peristaltic movements occur about every 30 minutes and several times per day there are larger contractions that help send the colonic contents towards and into the rectum. Food entering the stomach releases the hormone gastrin which enhances colonic motility.

The defaecation reflex is triggered by mass movements that stimulate stretch receptors in the rectum and this is sometimes referred to as the 'call to stool'. Relaxation of the muscles in the anal sphincters enable defaecation. As this is a voluntary activity, individuals can prevent defaecation and the urge will subside. One of the causes of constipation can be continually suppressing the call to stool – for example, if reliant on others for mobilising to the toilet.

Constipation

Causes of constipation are multi-faceted and include underlying issues such as:

- *faecal volume*: dietary fibre helps to 'bulk' up the stool so it is a larger volume and better stimulates peristalsis. Diets lacking in fibre result in smaller, less bulky stools with less peristalsis and predisposition to constipation;

(Continued)

145

(Continued)

- *transit time*: the amount of time taken for stools to travel through the colon depends on its muscle activity which can be affected by some disorders or medications. An increased transit time allows more water to be reabsorbed, thus causing smaller volume of faecal material and harder stools. In the extreme, bowel obstruction can be caused by a significant slowing of peristalsis, known as paralytic ileus. This can be caused by infections, mesenteric ischaemia, appendicitis, abdominal surgery and certain medications;
- *anatomical integrity*: a mass anywhere in the colon lumen, or sometimes outside it but causing pressure, can partially or completely block the passage of stools. This can cause longer transit time, changes in the characteristics of the stool (such as pencil-shaped, thin stools) or a bowel obstruction;
- *defaecation*: the rectum needs to become full to stretch the rectal wall and stimulate the sensing receptors, sending an impulse to nervous centres in the spinal cord to initiate the defecation reflex. Some disorders such as spinal cord injury or multiple sclerosis can impede the sensation and result in faecal incontinence or constipation;
- *medications*: there are a number of drugs that commonly cause constipation. NICE (2015c) guidelines for opioid prescribing in palliative care identify that constipation affects nearly all patients receiving strong opioid treatment and recommend laxative treatment for all patients initiating strong opioids. Laxatives themselves are a major cause of chronic constipation as, over time, frequent use can reduce intestinal muscle tone, resulting in an atonic, non-functioning colon.

We have briefly covered some of the main causes of constipation, but this isn't exhaustive so further information should be sought if this will be a common area for your future prescribing. The physiology of opioid-induced constipation is covered in further detail when we discuss treatment choices. Now that we have reviewed the basic anatomy, physiology and some causes of constipation, we can consider physical examination and what we are aiming to confirm through this.

Physical examination

As part of a thorough history, physical examination includes observing for signs of underlying causes, such as weight loss, cachexia or malnutrition which could indicate carcinoma, chronic conditions or depressive illness. You can observe for guarding and ask about pain and discomfort. Acute conditions such as obstruction can present with a tender abdomen, rigidity, guarding and absent bowel sounds. You may not be trained to perform full abdominal examination with palpation, etc., but should be able to listen for bowel sounds and check for visible abdominal distension and, with suitable training and experience, gently assess for masses or a palpable colon.

It is also recommended by CKS (NICE, 2020a) that a digital rectal examination (DRE) is undertaken to check for:

- anal fissure, haemorrhoids, skin tags, rectal prolapse, etc.;
- sphincter tone, rectal mass lesions, retained faecal mass, hardness of stool;
- leakage of stool, rectal or anal pain.

As DRE is invasive, informed consent is required and the practitioner needs to be competent in the procedure. There may be personal, gender-based, cultural, or other reasons why someone would decline a rectal examination so it is important to explain the procedure and why it is needed. In keeping with legal rulings around informed consent (Montgomery v Lanarkshire Health Board, 2015), it is also worth noting that risks of the examination versus not having it should be reasonably explained.

Embleton and Henderson (2020) noted that nurses don't always carry out digital rectal examinations when indicated, with many nurses citing lack of training as an influence on this practice. A portion of qualified nurses in their study were unaware they could undertake DRE (Embleton and Henderson, 2020) but the current proficiencies for pre-registration nursing students include *administer enemas and suppositories and undertake rectal examination and manual evacuation when appropriate* (NMC, 2018d, p26). Following a patient safety alert (NHS Improvement, 2018b), DRE training is an expectation of NHS employers and it can be undertaken by registrants who are able to demonstrate professional competence as per the NMC Code (2018a). It is also important to be aware of when DRE shouldn't be performed – for example, with rectal pain or bleeding, known abuse, recent surgery or trauma and various other reasons (RCN, 2019b). Activity 7.3 asks you consider whether DRE should be undertaken in this scenario with Mr Mo de Silva and what would influence your decision.

Activity 7.3   Decision-making: undertaking digital rectal examination

The history of Mo's presenting complaint indicates he may be constipated. Would you propose to undertake DRE and why? What might be some reasons to not undertake the examination in this example?

An example answer is provided at the end of the chapter.

Activity 7.3 asked you to identify reasons for and against undertaking DRE in this scenario. It is one example of a more invasive clinical examination that requires the practitioner to develop competence. Other examinations or investigations such as blood tests or abdominal exam may be applicable depending on the clinical history.

Investigations and tests

In this scenario, there were no clinical tests or further investigations that needed to be undertaken for Mo and the symptoms indicate an acute rather than chronic episode.

Diagnosis

We have gone through the stages of information-gathering combined with a knowledge of bowel function and evidence-based guidance to reach a working diagnosis of acute constipation. Mo has declined DRE so it is not possible to rule out faecal impaction, but the signs indicate a bowel obstruction is currently unlikely (although this can change, particularly without treatment). With constipation, the treatment can usually be based on the likely diagnosis in lieu of a definitive diagnosis after ruling out serious issues or red flag symptoms. CKS (NICE) suggest that no investigations are normally needed in an adult with functional constipation, where there is no suspected underlying cause. For Mo, opioid use is considered to be a secondary cause that requires consideration as part of the treatment plan, but not necessarily further investigation at this time.

Now that we have reached a working diagnosis for Mo, it is time to agree a treatment decision using CASE as a guide.

Making a CASE for treatment decisions

The aim of a shared decision is to agree the best course of action for that individual, improving adherence with the treatment regime and ideally a resolution of the problem. As per Figure 7.4, the CASE part of the consultation model focuses on a structured approach to the treatment decision by first looking at if a prescription is needed and, if so, its cost effectiveness, appropriateness, safety and effectiveness.

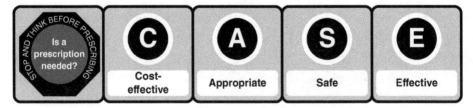

Figure 7.4   The CASE part of the RAPID-CASE consultation model

De-prescribing/alternatives to prescribing

The starting point is to question whether a prescription is required, or if de-prescribing is an option. In this scenario, opioid use may be the underlying cause, so the need for opioids should be assessed (NICE CKS, 2020a) and referral back to the GP considered. Opioids are recognised as one of the top ten dependency-forming medications (RCGP, 2019) and although seen as effective for short-term pain, there is little evidence to support their longer-term use for non-cancer pain (FPM, 2020). There is an increased risk of dependence and addiction if opioids are used for longer than three months (MHRA, 2020) and this can develop quickly, within just two to ten days of continuous use (NICE CKS, 2021e). NICE CKS (2020a) recommend managing the underlying cause of constipation by reducing or stopping drug treatments if appropriate, so referral or advice is indicated. Non-pharmacological self-care advice includes lifestyle measures such as a balanced diet with whole grains and fruits, and increasing fibre gradually, although the benefits may take weeks (NICE CKS, 2020a). Adequate fluid intake, increasing activity and exercise levels are also advisable if appropriate.

Cost effective

Prescribing options from the NPF are limited, and where products are not available, either from the NPF or local formularies, this may be due to their cost. In Mo's case, most of the commonly used products would be available and, with some exceptions, are relatively low cost, so the selection would largely be based on the most effective, appropriate and safest. One example exception is Naloxegol, which is a comparatively costly laxative (e.g. £1.84 per tablet versus £0.02 per Senokot tablet) approved for use by NICE (2015c) only in cases where opioid-induced constipation has not adequately responded to other laxatives (and not currently available in the NPF).

Appropriate

The BNF (JFC) and NICE CKS (2020a) indicate after lifestyle or dietary changes, bulk-forming laxatives are closest to natural dietary fibre. However, with Mo's clinical history, these would not be as suitable they aren't recommended for people taking constipating drugs (NICE CKS, 2020a). There are no other concerns in Mo's history, although safety considerations are applicable to anyone being prescribed certain laxatives.

Safe

Most laxatives are seen to be safe when used in moderation; a stepped approach is taken, although they are all contra-indicated with intestinal obstruction, perforation, paralytic ileus, Crohn's disease, or toxic megacolon. Specific contra-indications include avoiding: bulk-forming laxative when faecal impaction is suspected; lactulose in cases of galactosemia; or arachis oil enemas in people with a peanut allergy. There are various cautions to be aware of; co-danthramer or co-danthrusate has been found to have carcinogenic properties, so is limited to treating constipation for people who are terminally ill

(JFC, BNF). It is also important to note that excessive laxative use can lead to hypokalemia and longer-term issues with atonic bowel and chronic constipation.

Effective

The BNF provides an overview of how each main laxative works, while NICE CKS (2020a) include information on factors affecting laxative choice. Osmotic laxatives draw fluid into the bowel, or retain the fluid they were administered with, and increase bulk by bacterial fermentation. Macrogols also increase faecal bulk, but can additionally soften and rehydrate stools and are less dehydrating than other osmotics (RCN, 2019b). Some macrogol preparations are licensed to treat faecal impaction (JFC, BNF). Stimulant laxatives increase peristalsis so can cause abdominal cramps. For opioid-induced constipation, both a stool softener (or osmotic) and a stimulant laxative is advised (JFC, BNF). Docusate sodium is identified in the BNF as a stimulant laxative, but it is thought to also act as a softening agent, so may be a useful for people who have difficulty increasing their fluid intake.

The above provides an overview of the most common oral preparations for treating constipation, but rectal laxatives may also be indicated. These have the advantage of acting more quickly and predictably than oral preparations and work by softening or lubricating faeces, or act as a stimulant. The BNF also has three preparations identified as opioid receptor agonists for restricted use in people with opioid-induced constipation (mainly in palliative care), when other laxatives haven't worked. An outline of the pharmacology of these peripherally acting mu-opioid receptor antagonists (PAMRAs) is provided in Figure 7.5.

Opioids act as agonists at the three types of opioid receptors (mu, delta and kappa) to reduce pain (Ashelford *et al.*, 2019). Opioid (mu) receptors are also present in the bowel and action on these receptors causes gastrointestinal motility to be reduced. Naloxegol, Methylnaltrexone and Naldemedine selectively antagonise the peripheral opioid receptors. As antagonists, they block the effects of opioids (agonists) to help relieve constipation. These peripherally acting mu-opioid receptor antagonists

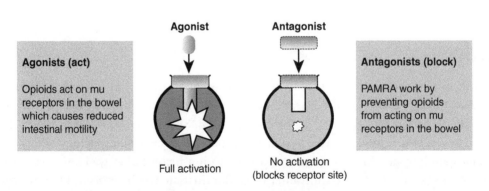

Figure 7.5 Agonist vs antagonist action on mu receptors

(PAMRAs) are in the BNF with some approved by NICE (2015c, 2020b) for specialist use, but not in the current edition of the NPF.

Now that we have reviewed the individual and treatment information, Activity 7.4 asks you to consider what to prescribe and influences on that decision.

Activity 7.4   Decision-making: what to prescribe

Mo would like treatment for his constipation. From a clinical perspective, what do you pro-pose as the best option for him and why?

An example answer is provided at the end of the chapter.

Activity 7.4 asked you to offer a solution as to which product(s) to prescribe and to con-sider the influences. This includes the person's perspective and priorities. Part of this process is to use summarisation to check the shared understanding of the presenting problem, diagnosis before providing information on the treatment options or recom-mendations, and follow-up care. The agreed plan should include lifestyle and self-care advice, a timeline for follow-up or monitoring and clear safety-netting advice. For Mo, you would either refer him (with his permission) or encourage him to seek advice for his back pain and opioid use. A reassessment of the presenting problem, or ensuring he is clear how to seek further support, is also advised. Providing information is both part of the shared decision-making and should frame your safety-netting advice. Activity 7.5 now asks you to identify information of pertinence about each of the preparations considered.

Activity 7.5   Critical thinking: what information?

You have considered the best clinical options to treat Mo's constipation. What does he need to know to aid informed choice and safe management afterwards? Some aspects of this include: how it works; the expected onset of action; when and how frequently he would need to take the preparation; any cautions or specific advice for administration. Use a for-mat like Table 7.1 to list the main laxative preparations. Included are two we have 'ruled out', but he may want an explanation of why these aren't recommended.

Laxative category	Information
Bulk-forming laxatives	
Faecal softeners	
Osmotic laxatives	
Stimulant laxatives	
PAMRAs	

Table 7.1   Laxative choice and information

No answer is provided for Activity 7.5 but this 'check list' can be used as a reminder of some of the points that potentially encourage concordance with the treatment and confidence in your advice. Have you provided information on:

- how the medicine works (at an appropriate level)?
- what to expect?
- how soon it should work?
- how well it should work (or how effective it should be)?
- any advice about administration?
- any precautions they should take?
- who to contact or what to do if they have concerns?
- what some of these concerns may be?
- what could be an adverse drug reaction, what to do and how to report it?
- how to store the product?
- when to stop taking?
- what to do with any leftover items at the end of the treatment?

Improper usage may cause the treatment to be ineffective, or prompt adverse effects, while incorrect storage can cause preparations to deteriorate. Persistence of the constipation, or worsening of symptoms such as abdominal discomfort, may require follow-up, although you would counsel that some laxatives include cramping as a side effect. Advising Mo would include expectations around the timeline, when to seek help if the problem persists or worsens, or what new symptoms require urgent attention.

Prescribing governance

At the end of the consultation, documentation is needed along with any onward referrals or notification of the wider multi-disciplinary team and clear communication with others in the team. As part of your continuing professional development, it is useful to reflect and record as you gain insight into the products you are prescribing. This is sometimes referred to as a 'personal formulary', which is essentially a template for noting details of items you have prescribed or are seeking to become comfortable with prescribing. These are available as mobile apps, or a document with headings such as:

- BNF/NPF section/drug class
- indications/condition being treated
- form/route/dose/dose interval (for the condition being treated)
- mode of action (how it works)
- contra-indications/cautions/side effects (common or important)

- interactions and the impact of these
- special instructions/advice/monitoring
- why this product? (guidelines/evidence source)

Other products in the NPF

We have outlined a systematic approach to one example product in the NPF, although recommend further exploration if you are new to prescribing for constipation. This same attention to detail and cognisance of influences on treatment decisions should be used for each area of prescribing practice you aim to develop. Activity 7.6 asks you to reflect on products from the NPF and identify which, if any, you are likely to prescribe in the future. This is followed by several activities using brief scenarios to encourage you to reflect about influences on prescribing. Some of these are likely to be outside your current scope of practice, but it is useful to identify where you will find reliable sources of information when dealing with unfamiliar circumstances.

Activity 7.6   Reflection: prescribing from the NPF

Table 7.2 lists the subsections of the NPF in column 1. Using this format, identify at least one specific item for each and describe these as fully as you can before looking them up. How likely are you to be prescribing these and what do you need to know? Although not applicable to all the preparations, you would want to identify for each product: indications; how it works; actions; time of onset; duration of action; side effect; routes and methods of administration; preparations and doses; treatment in special risk groups; cost; general advice or cautions.

1. NPF subsection	2. NPF item	3. Description
Laxatives		
Stoma care		
Analgesics		
Drugs for threadworms		
Appliances for diabetes		
Fertility products		
Urinary catheters		
Urinary disorders appliances		
Removal of ear wax		
Drugs for the mouth		

(Continued)

Table 7.2 (Continued)

1. NPF subsection	2. NPF item	3. Description
Emollients		
Barrier preparations		
Pruritic and skin conditions		
Parasiticidal preparations		
Disinfection and cleansing		
Wound management		
Local anaesthetics		
Neural tube defects		
Nicotine replacement therapy		

Table 7.2 Prescribing from the NPF

Activity 7.6 is aimed at getting you to think about the knowledge requirements for the products you may be prescribing. As covered in Chapter 2, prescribers from the NPF won't be able to prescribe for all of the indications listed in the BNF (e.g. mebendazole, malathion). In a similar way, ibuprofen can only be prescribed for the indications and at the doses stated in the Nurse Prescribers' Formulary. Taking the same approach as for the example of constipation, Activities 7.7 to 7.10 ask you to think critically about prescribing in these brief scenarios concerning the de Silva family. These cover five areas of the NPF and aim to encourage you to explore these to a greater depth. Along with a personal formulary, these are ways to guide your expanding scope of practice.

Activity 7.7 Critical thinking: practice scenario – candidiasis

Mo's wife Cath is normally well, but has not been feeling herself this past week or so, particularly since the concerns about her mother and being kept awake needing to feed six-week-old Milly in the night. You see her in baby clinic with the health visitor and she's complaining of breast discomfort. Milly has visible white patches on her tongue. What do you think may be the cause of these and what are the recommended treatment options?

Activity 7.7 asks you to think critically about the diagnoses and treatment options for Cath, who likely has a fungal skin infection, and her infant Milly, with oral thrush. Both of these conditions should be treated with a topical product – miconazole cream, for the skin infection and nystatin solution for the oral thrush. As per the NPF and BNF, oral miconazole is not licensed for infants under the age of four months due to a choking risk. It is worth noting that although fungal infections differ from mastitis (bacterial infection), they often follow antibiotic treatment but may also be a predisposing factor for recurrent mastitis (NICE CKS, 2021f). As mastitis can develop into sepsis, advice is needed regarding worsening signs, paracetamol use and awareness that it can mask a fever.

Activity 7.8   Critical thinking: practice scenario – eczema

Mo and Cath's son Sam had an episode of dry skin when he was an infant and they have recently noticed it seems to have returned, but is far worse. How would you assess this to make a diagnosis of childhood eczema? If the diagnosis of eczema is established, can all recommended treatment be prescribed from the NPF?

Activity 7.8 asks you to look at the process of diagnosing eczema versus a simple dry skin condition or other conditions that should be ruled out such as psoriasis, contact dermatitis, fungal infection or scabies (NICE CKS, 2021c). The correct diagnosis has significance for prescribing because although both dry skin conditions and eczema include emollients as first-line treatment, flare-ups of eczema may also require mild topical steroids (NICE CKS, 2021c). As these are not in the NPF, a referral to the GP, dermatologist or other prescriber may be needed. Considerations for practice include becoming familiar with assessing different skin types and conditions – for example, the presentations for people with naturally darker skin pigmentation may differ from pale skin. For eczema, the main signs such as dry skin, crusting, flakiness or thickening of the skin applies to all. The NICE CKS (2021c) note that while diagnostic criteria apply to all ages, social classes and ethnic groups, for *children of Asian, black Caribbean, and black African ethnic groups, atopic eczema can affect the extensor surfaces rather than the flexures, and discoid or follicular patterns may be more common.*

Activity 7.9   Critical thinking: practice scenario – lower leg wound

Cath tells you she has been dressing a small wound for her mum (Mrs Smith) since she moved in about six weeks ago. Cath is starting to worry because it doesn't seem to be improving. How would approach the assessment and planning for this wound?

Activity 7.9 concerns a commonly encountered issue for community nurses, as wound care comprises much prescribing and poses significant costs, with the care of people with chronic wounds found to account for nearly 50 per cent of community staff nurse time (Chapman *et al.*, 2017; Maybin *et al.*, 2016). Venous leg ulcers have an estimated prevalence of 0.1–0.3 per cent of the UK population (NICE CKS, 2021g) and wound care was provided for an estimated 3.8 million people in 2017 (Guest *et al.*, 2020); this is increasing each year. A wide variety of influences on decision-making are important for best practice and a structured approach to assessment and diagnosis is essential. For instance, it is necessary to assess for arterial disease as an urgent referral may be needed, or harm could occur if compression bandaging was applied inappropriately for someone with an arterial rather than venous leg ulcer. Pain is another issue of importance that sometimes gets overlooked. In a qualitative study of consultations for leg ulcers, Green *et al.* (2018b) found that the majority of practitioners neglected to raise the topic of pain or the emotional effects, with very few addressing those issues or the impact on daily life. Green *et al.* (2018b) emphasise that even highly skilled, experienced nurses may not proactively prompt discussions around the less 'clinical' aspects of care, or address these wider issues. To make a diagnosis in this instance a thorough assessment is required, including physical examination (e.g. doppler testing), pain assessment and consideration of the wider psycho-social factors that influence decision-making. CKS (NICE, 2021g) guidance alongside local assessment templates can help to guide and structure this, while Fletcher *et al.* (2019) additionally recommend using the *quality of life wound checklist* (Green *et al.*, 2018b) for a more rounded view of the issues and the impact on self-care.

Activity 7.10   Critical thinking: practice scenario – smoking cessation

Sana de Silva is 15 years old and has been secretly smoking for over a year. She is distraught as she doesn't want her parents to know, but has been having trouble quitting. She asks you to prescribe some chewing gum as one of her friends said it works well. How might you approach this situation?

Activity 7.10 concerns smoking cessation prescribing or advice for a teenager. As a professional, you would need to be working within your scope of practice, and within the remit of your scope and job description. For example, many areas commissioned separate smoking cessation services, removing the authority of their practitioners to prescribe for this. Where it is permitted, it may be a condition that you have attended training specific to smoking cessation. If it is established you are able to prescribe, the next step is to check if Sana is Gillick competent (CQC, 2018) and understands the implications and effects of a smoking cessation product.

Chapter summary

This chapter applied a structured approach to demonstrate the assessment of one example condition that can be prescribed for from the NPF. Although clinical decisions do not always involve a prescription, a structured approach is needed as illustrated through the discussion of some of the considerations when starting on your prescribing journey and the depth of knowledge required for safe and effective prescribing. This may include alternatives to a prescription such as advice for non-pharmacological treatments, reducing or stopping medicines or products the person can purchase to help aid cost effectiveness. Additional scenarios were used to prompt critical thinking around some of the other items you may be prescribing in the future within the context of your scope of practice. The use of a personal formulary to record your expanding knowledge base was recommended.

Activities: suggested answers and discussion points

Answer to Activity 7.2 Decision-making: identifying red and amber flag symptoms

Adults

- *Bowel obstruction*: this lack of ability for stool to move through the intestine can be partial or complete. Symptoms include: abdominal pain and distension, vomiting, inability to pass gas and possible dehydration. If untreated, the bowel may rupture, leak its contents and cause peritonitis and possible death (MedlinePlus, 2020a). There are a number of underlying causes.
- *Bowel perforation*: this is when a hole develops in the bowel causing leakage into the abdominal cavity. This can lead to peritonitis which is fatal without treatment. Symptoms include: chills, fever, severe abdominal pain, nausea, vomiting and shock (MedlinePlus, 2020b).
- *Faecal impaction*: this is when a large amount of hard stool is stuck in the rectum, normally in people who have been constipated for a period of time. It can lead to bowel obstruction. Impaction can also cause diminished rectal sensation and faecal incontinence that is mistaken for diarrhoea and treated incorrectly (RCN, 2019b).
- *Autonomic dysreflexia* (AD): a medical emergency unique to people with spinal cord injury and can lead to death if not treated. Signs and symptoms include: severe headache, flushing, sweating, blotchiness, hypertension. (For further information, please see RCN, 2019b.)
- May need urgent referral depending on circumstances (see RCN, 2019b) Undiagnosed rectal bleeding; undiagnosed diarrhoea, strangulated hernia (caused by straining).
- CKS (NICE, 2020a) recommend referral to a gastroenterologist or colorectal surgeon for specialist investigations and management if:
  - o a serious underlying cause such as colorectal cancer is suspected;
  - o an underlying secondary cause of constipation is suspected, which cannot be managed in primary care;
  - o symptoms persist or recur despite optimal management in primary care.
- It is also advisable to check the guidance on 'red flags' associated with gastrointestinal tract (lower) cancers – recognition and referral (NICE CKS, 2021h).

Children

There are several further concerns for children with signs of constipation, including some birth abnormalities and conditions, such as congenital aganglionic megacolon, anal stenosis, or neurological pathologies. Amber flags include developmental delay, concerns about wellbeing or possible safeguarding issues. Please see *Constipation in Children* (NICE CKS, 2020d) for further detail.

Answer to Activity 7.3 Decision-making: undertaking digital rectal examination

In the scenario, the purpose of a DRE would be to establish the presence, amount and consistency of faecal matter in the rectum. If the symptoms were likely to point to faecal impaction, the need for a suppository, or he was experiencing discomfort, the procedure and purpose would likely be justified and this would need to be explained.

However, depending on the history of his presenting complaint (e.g. short duration, not uncomfortable or painful) and his ability to articulate the information about the type and frequency of stool, DRE may not be needed. Another reason you might not perform a DRE is if there was a knowledge or skills gap, or if other factors complicated the scenario, such as rectal bleeding. There is clear guidance in the RCN (2019b) publication about when to not perform the procedure.

If you are skilled in DRE, it is indicated and safe to perform, he may still decline for personal reasons and this would need to be documented with decisions made using the best available information.

Answer to Activity 7.4 Decision-making: what to prescribe

While we have been able to exclude some items from consideration, the choice of product may still be influenced by your past experience(s), the person's preference or your local clinical formulary or guidelines, among other things. All of the products below are 'green' on most formularies, which indicates they are considered to be suitable for primary care prescribing, although you will need to check this in your practice area.

1. **No prescription**: although this may be managed by diet and stopping the opioids, depending on how uncomfortable he is, Mo may prefer a quicker solution and not want to stop his analgesia (or be reviewed for his back pain first).

2. **Rectal preparations**: As the constipation is reportedly of short duration, and there are no signs of faecal impaction, an oral remedy is likely preferred. Where DRE is declined, an enema is unlikely to be first choice unless the discomfort becomes more acute. When the drug action times are explained to Mo, he might opt for an enema if experiencing discomfort and not wanting to tolerate this much longer.

3. **Oral solutions** (excluding bulk-forming laxatives and PAMRAs):

    a. **Osmotics**: lactulose on its own in opioid-induced constipation may require high doses and is considered to be unpalatable, so macrogols are more favourable and less likely to cause cramping. Further, some are licensed for use in treating faecal impaction, giving Mo the option of increasing the dose if needed. Influences on this selection would be promoting his self-care, and ease of use, against the disadvantage of it taking two to three days to work and being slightly more costly than some of the other options. Local formularies may stipulate one brand over another to improve cost savings.

    b. **Stimulants**: senna or bisacodyl are two relative cheap and quick-acting options. However, they are more likely to cause cramping.

    c. **Combination**: to optimise independence another choice could be to prescribe both an osmotic and a stimulant (e.g. macrogol and senna); or docusate sodium capsules, which is thought to have both actions and is cost effective. However, docusate is unsuitable for people who need an oral solution as it is unpalatable and only fit for use in feeding tubes.

Further reading and useful websites

This chapter explored prescribing from the NPF. It is useful to become familiar with that publication alongside the British National Formulary and the Drug Tariff as these publications change regularly.

NICE BNF. https://bnf.nice.org.uk

NICE Nurse Prescribers' Formulary. https://bnf.nice.org.uk/nurse-prescribers-formulary/

NICE Nurse Prescribers' Formulary treatment summaries. https://bnf.nice.org.uk/nurse-prescribers-formulary/treatment-summary/

The Drug Tariffs vary between the countries and can be found at these links:

- National Health Service Drug Tariff for England and Wales. www.nhsbsa.nhs.uk/pharmacies-gp-practices-and-appliance-contractors/drug-tariff
- Health and Personal Social Services for Northern Ireland Drug Tariff. www.hscbusiness.hscni.net/services/2034.htm
- Scottish Drug Tariff. www.isdscotland.org/Health-topics/Prescribing-and-Medicines/Scottish-Drug-Tariff/

A good starting point for many clinical presentations is the NICE Clinical Knowledge Summaries. This has an A–Z guide that briefly covers common clinical conditions with the back-up of NICE guidelines and other reliable information.

NICE Clinical Knowledge Summaries (CKS). https://cks.nice.org.uk

Chapter 8

Preparation, proficiency and continuing professional development for prescribing

RPS Competency Framework for All Prescribers (2021a)

This chapter will address the following professional competencies:

- **Competency 7: Prescribe safely**
- **Competency 8: Prescribe professionally**
- **Competency 9: Improve prescribing practice**
- **Competency 10: Prescribe as part of a team**

NMC Future Nurse: Standards of Proficiency for Registered Nurses

This chapter will address the following platforms and proficiencies:

Platform 1: Being an accountable professional

At the point of registration, the registered nurse will be able to:

1.17 take responsibility for continuous self-reflection, seeking and responding to support and feedback to develop their professional knowledge and skills.

Chapter aims

After reading this chapter, you will be able to:

- explain accountability for maintaining competence as a prescriber;
- identify aspects of prescribing practice requiring continual development;
- outline a development plan, sources of support and information.

Introduction

You are a newly qualified registered nurse who is starting a new job in the community setting. You have observed from placements that nurses in this setting prescribe regularly. This makes you wonder if prescribing will be something you are expected to do, and how to develop your competence.

In line with updated standards (NMC, 2018b, 2019a), nurses and midwives are expected to have a proficient knowledge of pharmacology and be 'prescribing ready' at the preparing for the prescribing course prior to these standards may require to undertake some continuing professional development (CPD) to ensure their knowledge is what is expected of a registrant. Without the right preparation or facilitation, moving to a more advanced role can be challenging for new graduates. Those preparing for the prescribing course should become familiar with the RPS (2021a) competencies and ensure support mechanisms are in place within their employing organisation. Safe prescribing practice requires proficiency in assessment, diagnosis, evidence-based practice, pharmacological knowledge and a self-awareness of limitations (NMC, 2018e). The RPS (2021a) CFAP has now been adopted within the NMC (2018e) standards for prescribing programmes. However, the CFAP document was originally intended as a framework for continuing CPD.

Some principles are constant, but other aspects of prescribing, such as the research base, are continuously evolving. CPD is a professional requirement, necessary for safe practice, and involves keeping up to date within your current area of practice, as well as expanding that scope where appropriate. As a professional, you are expected to be aware of changes to guidelines, formularies, medicines advice and current 'best practice'. Ways to help address this requirement for maintaining currency of knowledge include identifying development needs, engaging with mandatory training and education through your employer, adhering to professional standards around revalidation (NMC, 2018a, 2019c) and seeking opportunities to keep your knowledge and skills up to date. A learning plan should encompass your ongoing development needs as a nurse or midwife registrant, as a specialist (in your particular area of expertise) and a prescriber.

This chapter starts with an outline of the preparation for transitioning to prescribing, followed by some background to the professional requirements for continuing professional development as a nurse and prescriber. The chapter discusses some of the challenges as well as benefits of CPD before exploring strategies and recommendations for optimising your learning time and gaining confidence as a prescribing practitioner.

Preparing for prescribing

Prescribing courses vary in intensity between community formulary prescribing (V100 or V150) and full formulary prescribing (V300) (as outlined in Chapter 1). Common to both is a time gap between completing the course and receiving your first prescription pad, which can affect confidence to start prescribing (Taylor and Bailey, 2017). Also, across all types of prescribers, there is an indication that some registered prescribers never prescribe, or do so very infrequently. A study from 2014 (Drennan *et al.*) found there was only a slight increase in overall prescribing by nurses after full formulary prescribing was legalised, with a rise from 1.1 per cent to 1.5 per cent of total items prescribed in primary care, although the data needs updating. A more recent study by Alghamdi *et al.* (2020) found a similar increase from 0.57 per cent in 2011–12 to 1.7 per cent in 2017–18, although this involved comparatively fewer nurse prescribers. The number of prescribers is steadily growing, with around 90,000 prescribers (NMC, 2020).

It is suggested not all prescribers are using their qualification or prescribing regularly, with various reasons for this proposed (Taylor and Bailey, 2017; McHugh *et al.*, 2020, Magowan, 2020). Noblet *et al.* (2017) noted in a systematic review that although many studies reported high job satisfaction and better autonomy for prescribers, key barriers included anxiety, increased job stress and time pressures. Common barriers for novice prescribers include increased workloads, low autonomy (e.g. through restrictive rules and policies), inadequate support or access to CPD (Noblet *et al.*, 2017; Casey *et al.*, 2020; Magowan, 2020). Burns (2021) noted a reduction in daily prescribing by pharmacists (from 51 per cent in 2019, to 44 per cent in 2020), which was largely attributed to job stress. Lim *et al.*'s (2018) study into doctors and nurses found they similarly experienced fear and anxiety as new prescribers, suggesting that expertise needs to be developed over time and with the support of senior colleagues. Facilitators of prescribing include having a defined area of competence, autonomy, access to data/support systems, ongoing education and CPD, organisational commitment, the support of pharmacists, other prescribers and clinical supervisors and using the competency framework (Lim *et al.*, 2018, Noblet *et al.*, 2017; Casey *et al.*, 2020; Burns, 2020; Magowan, 2020).

Some of the challenges to preparing to prescribe have been outlined along with some of the research into what helps to facilitate the practice of new prescribers. Activity 8.1 asks you to consider your current circumstances and the support available for when you attain the qualification.

Activity 8.1   Reflection: strategies for preparing to prescribe

You have successfully completed your community formulary nurse prescriber course and your NMC registration has been annotated with the prescribing qualification.

- What might be some of the barriers to starting out as a prescriber?
- What would help overcome some of the challenges?
- Where would you look for guidance, support and information?

Some example answers are provided at the end of the chapter.

Activity 8.1 asked you to identify some of the barriers and support mechanisms for preparing to prescribe in practice. This section looked at starting out as a prescriber, with access to CPD identified as one area which encourages safe prescribing practice. The next section discusses the health policy background to CPD and professional revalidation, before exploring strategies to embed this into your prescribing practice.

Background to continuing professional development requirements

Professional revalidation and continuing professional development (CPD) aim to protect the public from harm. Requirements for CPD, evidenced by the revalidation process (NMC, 2018a, 2019c), can be linked to two key inquiries into devastating health care failures: the *Bristol Royal Infirmary (BRI) Inquiry* and the 'Shipman Inquiry'. The *BRI Inquiry* (Kennedy, 2001) found practitioners were not required to keep their skills and knowledge up to date leading to the suggestion that all healthcare professionals should be contractually obliged to undergo appraisal, CPD and revalidation to ensure they remain competent to fulfil their job. In addition to ensuring a greater focus on the public interest by regulators, the report also recommended a duty of candour for professionals (Kennedy, 2001), although that was not enacted until after the Francis report (2013). The government's response included setting up an oversight body to strengthen and reform professional self-regulation processes, investing in CPD and encouraging the extension of revalidation to all professions (DoH, 2002b).

The Shipman Inquiry furthered this work, triggering a series of policy reforms aiming to ensure *trust, assurance and safety* (DoH, 2007b, c). The body providing oversight of the Nursing and Midwifery Council and other professional regulators was renamed the Professional Standards Authority (PSA) for health and social care and given wider powers over the years. In addition to inspecting the regulators, new powers include the legal authority to review 'fitness to practise' decisions and appeal decisions if they consider them to be insufficient for public protection (PSA, 2020). The overarching purpose of the regulators and the authority overseeing them is that of public protection. The Health and Social Care (Safety and Quality) Act [2015] defines their specific objective as follows:

a. *to protect, promote and maintain the health, safety and well-being of the public;*
b. *to promote and maintain public confidence in the professions regulated by the regulatory bodies;*
c. *to promote and maintain proper professional standards and conduct for members of those professions.*

While the PSA evaluates the performance of the NMC and other regulators, the NMC uses the Code (2018a) to assess the professionalism of its registrants, particularly when fitness to practise cases arise. The fours principles of prioritising people, practising effectively, preserving safety and promoting professionalism underpin public protection, guide practice and serve as a measure for assessing fitness to practise cases. Section 18 of the Code (NMC, 2018a) was introduced for fitness to practise cases concerning prescribing or medicines management.

We have discussed some of the background to professional regulation with its clearly defined objective of public protection. Activity 8.2 asks you to consider these processes as a member of the public who has concerns about the care being received by a friend.

Activity 8.2 Decision-making: reporting

Your former neighbour, Mrs James, is a life-long diabetic who is no longer able to self-inject insulin and was recently admitted to a care home. On a number of visits you have found she has clear signs of hyper- or hypo-glycemia. You have spoken to the registered nurse in charge on several occasions but they dismiss your concerns by saying she is just 'settling in' and probably not eating as regularly.

- How might you approach this before considering reporting it?
- Who might you contact if the situation continues or worsens?
- If it became necessary to report her to the NMC what would reassure you about the 'fitness to practise' process?

Some example answers are provided at the end of the chapter.

In Activity 8.2 you have considered potentially poor practice from your perspective as a member of the public. This next section discusses some of the more recent developments in professional regulation and the implications for your prescribing and continuing professional development.

First, do no harm

Despite continual modifications to professional regulation and healthcare policy, the Cumberlege (2020) report into medicines and medical devices safety opens with:

We have found that the healthcare system – in which I include the regulators and professional bodies, pharmaceutical and device manufacturers, and policymakers – is disjointed, siloed, unresponsive and defensive.

(Cumberlege, 2020, ppi–ii)

Aligned with best practice for individuals in your care, the report suggests listening to people as playing a pivotal role in spotting issues that may prompt safety concerns (Cumberlege, 2020). Recommendations of pertinence to prescribers include the MHRA (regulator of medicines and medical devices) putting people at the heart of its activity, and overhauling adverse event reporting and medical device regulation (Cumberlege, 2020). Another restructuring of professional regulation is in process (PSA, 2021a), and the Nursing and Midwifery Council has responded to past inspections by improving their fitness to practise processes to make them quicker and more transparent (PSA, 2021b). The most recent report (NMC, 2020) into fitness to practise cases identifies *prescribing and medicines management* as one of the top three categories where the most allegations were found proved, although most of these were for medicines management. This is a reminder of the need to stay updated to be aware of current best practice for the people in our care.

Professional regulation and continuing professional development

Some of the background and main influences on professional regulation including the need for CPD and revalidation have been outlined (NMC, 2018a, 2019c). With the ever-increasing emphasis on professional regulation and the continued expansion of prescribing, adequate support and practicable methods of CPD need to be established. Some of the specific professional standards influencing your prescribing practice include Section 6 of the Code regarding working in line with best evidence-based practice, and the specific imperative to keep your knowledge and skills current (NMC, 2018a). Section 13 concerns working within your area of competence and states that practitioners must *complete the necessary training before carrying out a new role* (NMC, 2018a, p13). In relation to prescribing, while the training itself addresses the RPS (2021a) competency framework, this must only be used in areas within your recognised area of clinical competence.

More specific to prescribing, Section 18 addresses your duty *to advise on, prescribe, supply, dispense or administer medicines within the limits of your training and competence, the law, our guidance and other relevant policies, guidance and regulations* (NMC, 2018a, p16). This encompasses the above need to only prescribe in areas of clinical competence as well as in line with evidence-based guidelines and other reliable information sources. Section 19 is also pertinent, with the need to be aware of, and reduce as far as possible, risks for harm. Prescribing clearly and appropriately, reporting incidents or adverse reactions and being aware of drug alerts or updates can all help to prevent medication errors. Related to each of these are the specific CPD requirements outlined in the Code (NMC, 2018a) to maintain your registration. These include the need to:

> 22.2 *keep to our prescribed hours of practice and carry out continuing professional development activities.*
>
> 22.3 *keep your knowledge and skills up to date, taking part in appropriate and regular learning and professional development activities that aim to maintain and develop your competence and improve your performance.*
>
> (NMC, 2018a, p.20)

One area of increased importance that requires additional development for many practitioners is that of remote prescribing. Nurses and midwives are normally with the person in their care, whereas with the COVID-19 pandemic it has become necessary to undertake remote consultations. The ability to safely assess people through remote means is a skill that needs to be developed and underpinned by core principles. Some resources to support this method of consultation can be found in the Further reading at the end of this chapter.

Continuing professional development as a prescriber

Despite the awareness of its vital importance by practitioners, employers, regulators, and researchers (Weglicki *et al.*, 2015), CPD for nurse and midwife prescribers has long been identified as inconsistent or challenging (Latter *et al.*, 2007; Ford and Otway, 2008; Carey and Courtenay, 2010; Nimmo *et al.*, 2017; Emrich-Mills *et al.*, 2019;

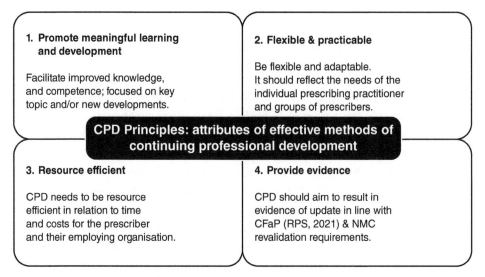

Figure 8.1 Principles for effective CPD

Paterson, 2019; Casey *et al.*, 2020; Wright and Jokhi, 2020). Time constraints and lack of organisational support are identified barriers to CPD (Latter *et al.*, 2007; Wainwright and Canning, 2008; Casey *et al.*, 2020). In view of the recognised need for CPD and intensifying governance arrangements, a robust strategy should be established to meet your ongoing CPD needs as a qualified prescriber. Despite a seeming gap between CPD standards and the ability to practically apply them, past experience and studies can be used to inform practice. Acceptable CPD strategies need commitment by prescribers as well as organisational support. Four principles of prescribing CPD are identified.

Methods of CPD

CPD requirements include a minimum of 20 hours of participatory learning within the 35 hours across three years (NMC, 2019c). Employing a range of strategies, such as participatory 'update' as well as online e-resources is most effective for the broad range of individual learning needs. These suggestions align with the four principles of prescribing CPD.

1. *Clinical update or study days*: NMC participatory learning (Principle 1, 4) These are delivered in different ways across organisations. Where a variety of topics or methods of delivery (such as webinars) are offered, flexibility is improved. Events can be organisation-wide or sourced externally and require mechanisms for evaluation and providing you with evidence of participation.

2. *Access to e-learning resources* (Principle 1, 3, 4) There is a wide variety of e-learning tools freely available to NHS staff and the public. These are excellent for flexibility and are largely resource-efficient. The limitations are around the support and protected time given to engaging with these resources. A selection of example resources for prescribing are provided at the end of the chapter, but there will be others of pertinence to your specific area of clinical expertise.

3. *Access to clinical supervision* (Principle 1, 3, 4) There is a consensus in most studies on CPD for prescribing that access to a supervisor or mentor is highly valuable. This could be the person who acted as your assessor, or an experienced and trusted colleague. This may be pre-established clinical supervision, but access to an experienced prescriber is beneficial. It is more likely to be an ad hoc arrangement, although a more structured 'preceptorship' period would be beneficial.

4. *Development of a professional portfolio* (Principle 1, 2, 3, 4) Keeping an ongoing record in the form of a portfolio using the RPS (2021a) framework will help to collate evidence of meeting revalidation and CPD requirements. It should also prompt reflection on practice which is a recognised learning strategy. The RPS (2021a) framework mentions using work-based tools to record ongoing competency as evidence can be through observed practice as well as reflection.

5. *Personal formulary* (Principle 1, 2, 4) Linked to the process of recording expanding knowledge through a portfolio, as discussed in Chapter 7, it is very useful to develop a 'personal formulary'. This is a way to remind of the core principle of needing

to know everything about a specific drug or product before prescribing it, and recording your expanding scope. Personal formularies are used by some prescribing programmes for assessment, and are available as documents or applications.

6. *Forms of evidence* Integral to a portfolio or as individual items is the use of feedback, reflective accounts, critical incidents, testimonies, observed consultations, case-based discussions or critical discussions with others.

This section outlined some practical strategies for meeting the learning needs of a developing prescriber. It is also useful to consider your progression from being a novice prescriber to that of a supervisor of others. To access prescribing courses, a degree of clinical expertise is required, and the learning journey to prescriber is part of that continuum. RPS (2021a) includes a competency statement around extending your practice to encouraging and supporting others with their prescribing practice. This may be periodic mentoring or clinical leadership in your area of expertise, but can also evolve into acting as a practice supervisor or assessor (NMC, 2018b) to facilitate others on their learning journey as a prescriber. The first steps involve growing your confidence as a safe and effective prescriber.

Activity 8.3 asks you to consider how you might approach a new role or responsibility as a prescriber in line with three key areas: your CPD requirements as a NMC registrant, within your specialist/defined area of practice and as a prescriber.

Activity 8.3 Critical thinking: expanding your prescribing practice – CPD planning

You are considered to be an expert practitioner in your defined area of practice who has been a prescriber for nearly one year. You have been asked to start prescribing in an area that is less familiar to you. What strategies would help to expand your scope of practice, minimise the risk of error and show evidence of developing competence? Identify a plan of action that takes into account CPD requirements in each of these three elements:

1. CPD requirements as a registered nurse or midwife (e.g. NMC revalidation);
2. CPD requirements as a 'specialist' (in your defined area of practice);
3. CDP requirements as a prescriber.

These three key areas are illustrated in Table 8.1 (CPD template).

1. CPD requirements and plan as a professional		
NMC requirements	How I intend to meet these	How this will be evidenced
20 hours participatory CPD activities		
35 hours CPD activities		

2. CPD requirements and plan as a specialist professional practitioner		
(e.g. paediatric nurse; memory clinic nurse; renal nurse; diabetic midwife; practice nurse; district nurse; health visitor)		
Professional and/or employer requirements	**How I intend to meet these**	**How this will be evidenced**
3. CPD requirements and plan as a prescriber		
Professional and/or employer requirements	**How I intend to meet these**	**How this will be evidenced**

Table 8.1 CPD template

Activity 8.3 asked you to consider how to approach expanding your practice, with a reference to CPD strategies. A model answer is provided at the end of the chapter, but this will be personalised to your area of practice and specific job role.

Chapter summary

This chapter considered your accountability and methods by which to keep up to date as a prescriber. It is recommended that as part of your transition to an active prescriber, you outline a development plan and identify the sources of support and information required for your safe and effective prescribing practice. While it is important to gain in confidence as a prescribing practitioner, you should also recognise there will always be things to learn. It is vital that you reflect on your practice to identify areas for further learning. This awareness extends to the need to consider diagnoses and treatments outside your current knowledge, and will ultimately help reduce the risks of complacency and prescribing errors.

Prescribing by nurses has come a long way since 1986 when Baroness Cumberlege (2003) witnessed fully competent nurses waiting for GPs to sign prescriptions that they may have written themselves. Having seen the gradual expansion of prescribing, Cumberlege (2003, p12) commented that it is *not only about user satisfaction and clinical practice but also power and professional territory*. To uphold the reputation of the profession and this hard-fought autonomy, it is incumbent on nurses and midwives to use great care and attention when deploying these prescribing powers.

Activities: suggested answers and discussion points

Answer to Activity 8.1 Reflection: strategies for preparing to prescribe

Some of the barriers as a prescriber have been outlined in the research, and you may find these resonate with your practice setting. For example, time pressures and concerns about additional workload are widespread. Addressing these depends on the individual circumstances, but is broadly linked to how supported and confident you feel in decision-making. Employer policies and formularies may seem restrictive to experienced prescribers, but are important places to start on the prescribing journey, along with electronic decision-support tools as mentioned in Chapter 4. Additionally, guidance and support should be sought from experienced prescribers, including those who have provided assessment and supervision while you were achieving the competencies. The RPS (2021a) competency framework for prescribers is a way to review your progress and identify areas for further development. When you gain more confidence as a prescriber, it is also helpful to review prescribing analysis and cost data.

Answer to Activity 8.2 Decision-making: reporting

How you approach any concerns about practice should be guided by the NMC Code (2018a), which is clear about the need to raise these if a person is at risk. Although this isn't a colleague you are directly working with, some of the principles in Section 8 and 9 of the Code may be applicable, at least while you are assessing the situation. Where the situation continues or worsens, particularly if risk of harm is involved and reporting to the manager has failed, the CQC or NMC can be contacted. While it can be a matter of opinion as to what would be reassuring about the 'fitness to practise' process, both for those who refer a practitioner and for those who are subject to investigation, a quick resolution is desirable. The process also needs to be fair and robust to achieve its aim of public protection.

Answer to Activity 8.3 Critical thinking: expanding your prescribing practice – CPD planning

It is useful to have a CPD plan, whether for a change of scope of practice, or to identify methods of support post-qualification. An example is provided below in Table 8.2, which outlines these three key elements:

1. CPD requirements as a registered nurse or midwife (e.g. NMC revalidation);

2. CPD requirements as a 'specialist' (in your defined area of practice);

3. CDP requirements as a prescriber.

1. CPD requirements and plan as a professional		
NMC requirements	**How I intend to meet these**	**How this will be evidenced**
20 hours participatory CPD activities	Clinical supervision sessions; study days	Reflective pieces for portfolio
35 hours CPD activities	Independent learning; online course; conference attendance, etc.	Reflective pieces and CPD learning log
2. CPD requirements and plan as a specialist professional practitioner		
(e.g. paediatric nurse; memory clinic nurse; renal nurse; diabetic midwife; practice nurse; district nurse; health visitor). May be employer led		
Professional and/or employer requirements	**How I intend to meet these**	**How this will be evidenced**

E.g. paediatric nurse: mandatory calculations update	Online learning	Mandatory calculations test
E.g. palliative care nurse: update re. best practice and current treatments	Identify a palliative care consultant for peer support and clinical supervision	Reflective pieces; learning log
Updates re. new guidelines	Specialist study days	Reflective pieces; learning log; PDR
3. CPD requirements and plan as a prescriber		
Professional and/or employer requirements	**How I intend to meet these**	**How this will be evidenced**
E.g. attendance at CPD study days	Attend a selection of Trust-provided CPD study days	Reflective pieces; learning log/record
Preceptorship	Identify a qualified prescriber for peer support and clinical supervision	
Keep up to date with drug interactions, alerts, etc.	Subscribe to MHRA alerts; subscribe to automated updates on prescribing	Learning log; performance review
Accessing prescribing analysis and cost data	Various ways to access; Walker et al. (2019) discuss how a database for practitioners has changed prescribing practice	

Table 8.2   Example CPD plan using a template

Further reading and useful websites

We explored keeping up to date with prescribing generally, as well as remote prescribing. These resources are focused on prescribing or medicines, but it is also important to find CPD resources for your specialist or specific area(s) of prescribing practice.

Medicines management and prescribing

The NMC withdrew its medicines management standards in 2019, so resources to support this theme can be found on the RCN website that hosts a repository for pertinent resource links and information. https://www.rcn.org.uk/clinical-topics/medicines-management

The Royal Pharmaceutical Society also addresses aspects of medicines management with its useful Medicines Optimisation Hub. https://www.rpharms.com/resources/pharmacy-guides/medicines-optimisation-hub

It is worth exploring the NICE quality standard relating to medicines optimisation as this identifies expectations: https://www.nice.org.uk/guidance/QS120

The Royal Pharmaceutical Society has also published guidance on the handling of medicines and, in collaboration with the RCN, on medicines administration. Both of these can be found at the same link.

- Royal Pharmaceutical Society (2018) *Professional Guidance on the Safe and Secure Handling of Medicines*
- Royal Pharmaceutical Society and Royal College of Nursing (2019) *Professional Guidance on the Administration of Medicines in Health Care Settings*

https://www.rpharms.com/recognition/setting-professional-standards/safe-and-secure-handling-of-medicines

We explored keeping up to date with prescribing by looking at prescribing patterns. You may wish to explore the database open prescribing.net. https://openprescribing.net

Remote prescribing

Pre-COVID-19 the NMC and other regulators or healthcare organisations worked together to publish core principles for good practice in remote consultations and prescribing. The aim was to help protect patient safety for online or telephone-based access to potentially harmful medications. *The jointly-agreed* High level principles for good practice in remote consultations and prescribing *sets out the good practice expected of healthcare professionals when prescribing medication online* (NMC, 2019b).

Nursing and Midwifery Council (2019b) High Level Principles for Good Practice in Remote Consultations and Prescribing. https://www.nmc.org.uk/standards/standards-for-post-registration/standards-for-prescribers/useful-information-for-prescribers/

However, while the principles are necessarily cautious, the increased need for remote contact prompted a number of resources aimed at practitioners involved with remote consultation. Resources are accessible from the several professional colleges including the Royal College of Nursing (2020a), *Prescribing Safely Under COVID-19*. This page also contains links to further resources to support safe prescribing.

https://www.rcn.org.uk/clinical-topics/medicines-management/covid-19-remote-prescribing

The General Medical Council has updated its prescribing guidance to reflect the move to remote prescribing during and post-COVID-19. Although aimed at medical practitioners, the guidance can be very helpful for all prescribers, outlining core principles in different situations.

GMC (2021) *Good Practice in Prescribing and Managing Medicines and Devices.* https://www.gmc-uk.org/ethical-guidance/ethical-guidance-for-doctors/good-practice-in-prescribing-and-managing-medicines-and-devices

Glossary

Absorption   when referring to medicines, is a pharmacokinetic parameter that refers to the way a drug is absorbed from a pharmaceutical formulation into the bloodstream.

Active metabolite   results when a drug is metabolised by the body into a modified form which continues to produce effects in the body.

Active tubular secretion   many drugs are eliminated by the kidney by tubular secretion. If this is not passive and needs energy, it is called active tubular secretion.

ADME   Absorption, Distribution, Metabolism, Elimination

ADR   adverse drug reaction

Adverse events/adverse drug reactions   these are reactions to medicines that were unexpected, unintended and may cause harm to the patient.

Agonist   an agonist is a compound that can bind to and cause activation of a receptor.

Antagonist   an antagonist is a compound that has the opposite effect of an agonist. It decreases the activation of a receptor by binding and blocking neurotransmitters.

Augmented (Type A) classification of an adverse drug reaction   this is a type of adverse drug reaction that is usually dose-related, is correlated with the drug's pharmacological action, are largely predictable. Although mortality is low, morbidity may be high. They are generally detected during clinical trials.

Bioavailability   the proportion of any taken medicine that reaches the systemic circulation. Usually referred to on a 0–1 scale.

Biotransformation   processes which result in alteration of the original compound.

Bizarre (Type B) adverse drug reactions   this is part of the classification of adverse drug reactions which is not predictable and has the potential for mortality. As this is not as common as Type A they are not usually detected during clinical trials.

Blood brain barrier   this is a network of blood vessels and tissue that is made up of closely spaced cells and helps keep harmful substances from reaching the brain.

BNF   British National Formulary

Cautions   The BNF uses the term cautions to help minimise harm and drug safety. Caution is used to help assess the risk of using a drug in a particular patient. The drug can still be used if a safer preparation cannot be found.

Co-morbidities   having more than one condition to treat.

Contra-indications   these are far more restrictive than cautions and mean that the drug should be avoided in patients where the drug is contra-indicated.

Cytochrome P450   this is a group of enzymes which play a key role in the metabolism of many drugs.

CYP450 see cytochrome P450

Diffusion   the method by which most drugs (and other substances) cross into and out of cells. Areas of high concentration move to areas with lower concentration until there is a balance. This passive diffusion is the main way drugs are distributed.

Distribution (pre- and post-liver)   drugs are absorbed and pass to the liver via the hepatic portal vein. They may then be metabolised to a greater or lesser degree and pass into the systemic circulation. Some metabolites may reach the gall bladder to be re-secreted into the gut.

DOAC   direct oral anticoagulant

Drug interactions   drug interactions can occur between two or more drugs taken together and may enhance or cancel out the effects of one or all of the drugs. They can be pharmacokinetic or pharmacodynamic in nature. Food and alcohol may also interact with medicines.

Elimination   metabolism and excretion together are sometimes referred to as elimination.

Enteral   enteral administration is food or drug administration via the human gastrointestinal tract. This contrasts with parenteral nutrition or drug administration.

Enzyme inducer   enzymes can break down drugs. Enzyme inducers enhance the production of liver enzymes which break down drugs. This means less drug will be available for action.

Enzyme inhibitor   these are, for example, drugs which can block the metabolism of another drug which means more of that drug remains within the system, which could lead to toxicity.

Enzymes   are catalysts in living organisms regulating the rate at which chemical reactions proceed without themselves being altered in the process.

Excretion   is a process in which metabolic waste is eliminated from an organism. In vertebrates, this is primarily carried out by the lungs, kidneys and skin.

First-pass metabolism   absorbed drugs (or other material) passes to the liver via the hepatic portal vein where it can be metabolised. This first metabolism is known as first pass. In a circulatory system, the material will pass through the liver again.

Free drugs   many drugs are attached to proteins in the plasma to be distributed. Some that are not bound to proteins are called free drugs. Only free drugs can have an action.

GI system   the gastrointestinal system

Glomerular filtration   is the renal process whereby fluid in the blood is filtered across the capillaries of the glomerulus.

G6PD deficiency   a genetic condition leading to a deficiency of glucose-6-phosphate dehydrogenase.

Half-life   is the time required to reduce the plasma concentration of a drug to half of its original value.

Hypoalbuminaemia   is where the level of albumin in the blood is low. This can have an effect on the distribution of drugs within the systemic circulation.

Ligand   any substance (exogenous/endogenous) that binds to a receptor.

Lipid-soluble   the ability of a molecule to dissolve in lipids (fats). Most drugs are lipid-soluble, so are able to diffuse across cell membranes.

Metabolism   the body's action on, for example, drugs. There are three aspects of metabolism: activation of an inactive drug, production of active drug from an already active drug or inactivation of active drugs.

Metabolite   the product of the metabolic process. Some will be active.

MHRA   Medicines and Healthcare Products Regulatory Agency

NICE   National Institute for Health and Care Excellence

NMC   Nursing and Midwifery Council

Parenteral   taken into the body or administered in a manner other than through the digestive tract, as by intravenous or intra-muscular injection.

Partial antagonist   binds to and activates a receptor but is not able to elicit the maximum possible response that is produced by a full agonist.

Passive tubular reabsorption   happens in the kidney nephrons. Energy is not required and the body can reabsorb ions such as sodium passively as required.

Pharmacodynamics   the effect the drug has on the body.

Pharmacology   is a science that looks at the composition, effects and uses of drugs.

Pharmacokinetics   how the body processes a drug.

Pharmacovigilance   pharmacovigilance is the science and activities relating to the detection, assessment, understanding and prevention of adverse effects or any other medicine/vaccine-related problem.

Phase 1 or Phase 2 reactions   these are part of metabolism. Phase 1 reactions are, oxidation, reduction and hydrolysis and usually form more reactive products, sometimes toxic, whereas Phase 2 reactions from conjugates usually form inactive and readily excretable products.

PIL   patient information leaflet

Placental barrier   composed of both maternal and foetal tissue, which acts as another internal *barrier* that can protect the development of embryo.

Polar   (also known as water soluble) these refer to molecules that have a slight positive charge on one side and a slight negative charge on the other. The charge creates difficulty for diffusing across a membrane. Water molecules are polar, so other polar molecules can normally dissolve in water and are known as hydrophilic. In contrast, non-polar molecules are said to be hydrophobic and, most often, lipophilic, or lipid-soluble.

Glossary

Prodrugs   pharmacologically inactive substance that is converted in the body (such as by enzymatic action) into a pharmacologically active drug.

Product   a metabolite which is formed following metabolism by the cytochrome P450 enzymes.

Protein-bound   drugs bind to proteins in the circulatory system after passing through the liver. Only free drugs can have an action on the body.

RPS   Royal Pharmaceutical Society

Steady state   in pharmacokinetics, steady state refers to the situation where the overall intake of a drug is in equilibrium with its elimination.

Substrate   a drug or other substance which is metabolised by the cytochrome P450 enzymes.

Systemic   means affecting the whole body. It is in contrast with topical or local.

Topical   a *topical medication* is a *medication* that is applied to a particular place on or in the body. Most often *topical* administration *means* application to body surfaces.

Toxicity   refers to how *poisonous* or harmful a substance can be. It can occur from a *drug* overdose or from the intake of a prescribed medication.

Water soluble   means the medicine or substance can dissolve in water.

Bibliography

Acheson, D (1988) *Public Health in England: The Report of the Committee of Inquiry into the Future Development of the Public Health Function.* London: HMSO.

Acheson, D (1998) *Independent Enquiry into Inequalities in Health.* London: HMSO.

Age of Legal Capacity (Scotland) Act 1991. Available at: https://www.legislation.gov.uk/ukpga/1991/50

Airedale NHS Trust v Bland [1993] AC 789. Available at: http://www.e-lawresources.co.uk/Airedale-N-H-S–Trust-v-Bland.php

Alberts, B, Johnson, A, Lewis, J, *et al.* (2002) *Molecular Biology of the Cell* (4th edn). New York: Garland Science. Blood Vessels and Endothelial Cells. Available at: https://www.ncbi.nlm.nih.gov/books/NBK26848/

Alghamdi, SSA, Hodson K, Deslandes P, Gillespie D, *et al.* (2020) Prescribing trends over time by non-medical independent prescribers in primary care settings across Wales (2011–2018): a secondary database analysis. *BMJ Open; 10*:e036379. doi:10.1136/bmjopen-2019-036379

Ali, M (2017) Communication skills 1: benefits of effective communication for patients. *Nursing Times [online], 113*(12), 18–19.

Allam, J, Bowen, G, Goodeve, M, Manu, C, Meally, H, Mitchell, L, Russell, D and Sharpe, A (2018) Best practice recommendations for the implementation of a DFU treatment pathway. *Wounds UK* [online]. Available at: https://www.wounds-uk.com/resources/details/best-practice-recommendations-for-the-implementation-of-a-dfu-treatment-pathway

Allen, I (2021) *Maintaining the COVID-19 Vaccines Cold Chain.* Available at: https://www.sps.nhs.uk/articles/maintaining-the-covid-19-vaccines-cold-chain/

Alper, B and Haynes, R (2016) EBHC pyramid 5.0 for accessing preappraised evidence and guidance. *BMJ Evidence-Based Medicine* [online]; *21*:123–5. Available at: https://ebm.bmj.com/content/21/4/123

Ashelford, S, Raynsford, J and Taylor, V (2019) *Pathophysiology and Pharmacology in Nursing* (2nd edn). London: Sage.

Baird, B, Boyle, T, Chauhan, K, Heller, A and Proce, C (2020) *How to Build Effective Teams in General Practice* [online]. Available at: https://www.kingsfund.org.uk/publications/effective-teams-general-practice

Barnett, N, Athwal, D and Rosenbloom, K (2011) Medicines-related admissions: you can identify patients to stop that happening. *The Pharmaceutical Journal* [online]. Available at: https://www.pharmaceutical-journal.com/learning/learning-article/medicines-related-admissions-you-can-identify-patients-to-stop-that-happening/11073473.article

Barr, J and Dowding, L (2012) *Leadership in Health Care* (2nd edn). London: Sage.

Beauchamp, TL and Childress, JF (2019) *Principles of Biomedical Ethics* (8th edn). New York: Oxford University Press.

Bentley, J, Heard, K, Collins, G and Chung, C (2015) Mixing medicines: how to ensure patient safety. *The Pharmaceutical Journal*, 14 April. Available at: https://pharmaceutical-journal.com/article/ld/mixing-medicines-how-to-ensure-patient-safety

Black, J and Simende, A (2020) Ten top tips: assessing darkly pigmented skin. *Wounds International* [online]. Available at: https://www.woundsinternational.com/resources/details/ten-top-tips-assessing-darkly-pigmented-skin

Bolam v Friern HMC [1957] 1 WLR 582. Available at: http://www.e-lawresources.co.uk/Bolam-v–Friern-Hospital-Management-Committee.php

Bolitho v City and Hackney Health Authority [1997] AC 232. Available at: https://www.lawteacher.net/cases/bolitho-v-hackney.php

Bolton, D (2015) Two nurses jailed for neglect after faking patients' blood glucose test results. *The Independent*. Available at: https://www.independent.co.uk/news/uk/home-news/bridgend-wales-nurses-jailed-for-neglect-a6773431.html

British Medical Journal (BMJ) Alerts. https://www.bmj.com/alerts

Burchum, JR, Rosenthal, LD, Jones, BO, Neumiller, JJ and Lehne, RA (2016) *Lehne's Pharmacology for Nursing Care* (9th edn). St Louis, MI: Elsevier/Saunders.

Burns, C (2021) Dip in number of pharmacists who prescribe daily. *The Pharmaceutical Journal*, October. Available at: https://pharmaceutical-journal.com/article/news/dip-in-number-of-pharmacists-who-prescribe-daily

Burton Shepard, A (2019) To prescribe or not to prescribe: enhancing safety in remote prescribing. *Journal of Prescribing Practice* [online], *1*(3). Available at: https://doi-org.ezproxy.derby.ac.uk/10.12968/npre.2018.16.3.134

Care Quality Commission (CQC) (2018) *Nigel's Surgery 8: Gillick Competency and Fraser Guidelines*. Available at: https://www.cqc.org.uk/guidance-providers/gps/nigels-surgery-8-gillick-competency-fraser-guidelines

Care Quality Commission (CQC) (2019) *Nigel's Surgery 19: Patient Group Directions (PGDs)/Patient Specific Directions (PSDs)*. Available at: https://www.cqc.org.uk/guidance-providers/gps/nigels-surgery-19-patient-group-directions-pgds-patient-specific-directions

Care Quality Commission (CQC) (2021) *Reporting Medicine Related Incidents*. Available at: https://www.cqc.org.uk/guidance-providers/adult-social-care/reporting-medicine-related-incidents

Carey, N and Courtenay, M (2010) An exploration of the continuing professional development needs of nurse prescribers and nurse supplementary prescribers who prescribe medicines for patient with diabetes. *Journal of Clinical Nursing, 19*(1–2): 208–21.

Carter, L (2018) Consultation models in practice. *GP Online [online]*. Available at: https://www.gponline.com/consultation-models-practice/article/988629

Casey, M, Rohde, D, Higgins, A, Buckley T, *et al.* (2020) 'Providing a complete episode of care': A survey of registered nurse and registered midwife prescribing behaviours and practices. *Journal of Clinical Nursing, 29*: 152–62. Available at: https://doi.org/10.1111/jocn.15073

Cathala, X and Moorley, C (2020) Performing an A–G patient assessment: a practical step-by-step guide. *Nursing Times, 116*(1): 53–5.

Cavanagh, S (2020) An introduction to PGDs: definitions and examples of use. *Specialist Pharmacy Service.* Available at: https://www.sps.nhs.uk/articles/what-is-a-patient-group-direction-pgd/

Centre for Evidence-based Medicine (CEBM) (2021) *Critical Appraisal Tools.* Available at: https://www.cebm.net/2014/06/critical-appraisal/

Centre for Reviews and Dissemination (2021) https://www.york.ac.uk/crd/

Chamberlain-Salaun, J, Mills, J and Usher, K (2013) Terminology used to describe health care teams: an integrative review of the literature. *Journal of Multidisciplinary Healthcare, 6*: 65–74.

Chapman, H, Kilner, M, Matthews, R, White, A, Thompson, A, Fowler-Davis, S and Farndon, L (2017) Developing a caseload classification tool for community nursing. *British Journal of Community Nursing, 22*(4): 192–6.

Charles, A (2021) *Integrated Care Systems Explained: Making Sense of Systems, Places and Neighbourhoods* [online]. Available at: https://www.kingsfund.org.uk/publications/integrated-care-systems-explained

Children Act 1989. Available at: http://www.legislation.gov.uk/ukpga/1989/41/contents

Cochrane (2020) *About Cochrane Reviews.* Available at: https://www.cochranelibrary.com/about/about-cochrane-reviews

Cochrane Clinical Answers. Available at: https://www.cochranelibrary.com/cca/about

Cochrane Evidence Summaries. Available at: https://www.cochrane.org/evidence

Cochrane Library. Available at: https://www.cochranelibrary.com

Conforth, A (2013) Holistic wound assessment in primary care. *British Journal of Community Nursing, 18*(12).

Conn, R, Kearney, O, Tully, M, Shields, M, *et al.* (2019) What causes prescribing errors in children? Scoping review. *BMJ Open.* Available at: https://bmjopen.bmj.com/content/9/8/e028680.long

Council Directive 92/26/EEC of 31 March 1992 concerning the classification for the supply of medicinal products for human use. Available at: https://www.legislation.gov.uk/eudr/1992/26/adopted#

Courtenay, M and Chater, A (2021) Antimicrobial stewardship: a competency framework to support the role of nurses. *Primary Health Care.* Available at: http://orca.cf.ac.uk/137079/

Criminal Justice and Courts Act 2015 Available at: https://www.legislation.gov.uk/ukpga/2015/2/contents/enacted

Cullum, N, Buckley, H and Dumville, J (eds) (2016) Wounds research for patient benefit: a 5–year programme of research. Programme Grants Appl Res 4(13). Southampton (UK). *NIHR Journals Library*. Available at: https://www.ncbi.nlm.nih.gov/books/NBK379923/

Cumberlege, J (2003) A triumph of sense over tradition: the development of nurse prescribing. *Nurse Prescribing*, *1*(1): 10–14. Available at: https://doi.org/10.12968/npre.2003.1.1.11180

Cumberlege, J (2020) '*First Do No Harm*'. Independent Medicines and Medical Devices Safety Review, chaired by Baroness Julia Cumberlege. Available at: https://www.immdsreview.org.uk/Report.html

Dalton, D and Williams, N (2014) Building a Culture of Candour: A Review of the Threshold for the Duty of Candour and of the Incentives for Care Organisations to be Candid. Available at: http://www.rcseng.ac.uk/policy/documents/CandourreviewFinal.pdf

Day, P, Gould, J and Hazelby, G (2020) A public health approach to social isolation in the elderly. *Journal of Community Nursing*, *34*(3). Available at: https://www.jcn.co.uk/journals/issue/06-2020/article/a-public-health-approach-to-social-isolation-in-the-elderly

Denness, C (2013) What are consultation models for? Available at: http://journals.sagepub.com/doi/full/10.1177/1755738013475436

Department for Constitutional Affairs (DCA) (2007) *The Mental Capacity Act 2005 Code of Practice*. Issued by the Lord Chancellor on 23 April in accordance with sections 42 and 43 of the Act [online]. Available at: https://www.gov.uk/government/publications/mental-capacity-act-code-of-practice

Department of Health (DoH) (1989) *Report to the advisory group on Nurse Prescribing* (Crown report). London: DoH.

Department of Health (DoH) (1991) *Nurse prescribing – final report: a cost benefit study* (Touche Ross report). London: DoH.

Department of Health (DoH) (1998a) *Report on the Supply and Administration of Medicines under Group Protocols* HSC1998/051. London: DoH.

Department of Health (DoH) (1998b) *Quality in the New NHS*. London: DoH.

Department of Health (DoH) (1999) *Review of prescribing, supply and administration of medicines. Final report* (Crown report II). London: HMSO. Available at: https://webarchive.nationalarchives.gov.uk/+/http://www.dh.gov.uk/en/Publicationsandstatistics/Publications/PublicationsPolicyAndGuidance/DH_4077151

Department of Health (DoH) (2002a) *Liberating the talents: helping primary care trusts and nurses to deliver the NHS plan*. London: DoH.

Department of Health (DoH) (2002b) *Learning from Bristol: the Department of Health's response to the report of the Public Inquiry into children's heart surgery at the Bristol Royal Infirmary 1984–1995*. Available at: https://www.gov.uk/government/publications/the-department-of-healths-response-to-the-report-of-the-public-inquiry-into-childrens-heart-surgery-at-the-bristol-royal-infirmary

Department of Health (DoH) (2004) *Prescribing: an essential skill of the nurse of the future.* London: DoH.

Department of Health (DoH) (2005) *An evaluation of extended formulary nurse prescribing.* London: DoH/University of Southampton.

Department of Health (DoH) (2006a) *Improving Patients' Access to Medicines: A Guide to Implementing Nurse and Pharmacist Independent Prescribing within the NHS in England.* London: DoH.

Department of Health (DoH) (2006b) *Safety First.* London: DoH.

Department of Health (DoH) (2006c) *Modernising Nursing Careers: Setting the Direction, CNOs Directorate.* London: DoH.

Department of Health (DoH) (2007a) *Nurse Independent Prescribing.* London: DoH.

Department of Health (DoH) (2007b) *Trust, assurance and safety: the regulation of health professionals in the 21st century.* Available at: https://www.gov.uk/government/publications/trust-assurance-and-safety-the-regulation-of-health-professionals-in-the-21st-century

Department of Health (DoH) (2007c) *Learning from tragedy, keeping patients safe: Overview of the Government's Action programme in response to the recommendations of the Shipman Inquiry.* London: HMSO. Available at: https://www.gov.uk/government/publications/overview-of-the-governments-action-programme-in-response-to-the-recommendations-of-the-shipman-inquiry

Department of Health (DoH) (2009) *Making the Connections: Using Healthcare Professionals as Prescribers to Deliver Organisational Improvements.* London: DoH. Gateway Reference 11538

Department of Health (DoH) (2010) *Mixing of medicines prior to administration in clinical practice: medical and non-medical prescribing.* London: DoH.

Department of Health and Social Care (DHSC) (2015a) *Mental Health Act 1983: Code of Practice Presented to Parliament pursuant to section 118 of the Mental Health Act 1983.* Available at: https://www.gov.uk/government/publications/code-of-practice-mental-health-act-1983

Department of Health and Social Care (DHSC) (2015b) *Mental Health Act 1983: Reference Guide.* Available at: https://www.gov.uk/government/publications/mental-health-act-1983-reference-guide

Department of Health and Social Care (DHSC) (2018a) *The Report of the Short Life Working Group on Reducing Medication-related Harm.* Available at: https://www.gov.uk/government/publications/medication-errors-short-life-working-group-report

Department of Health (2018b) *Working Together to Safeguard Children: A Guide to Inter-Agency Working to Safeguard and Promote the Welfare of Children.* [online]. Available at: https://www.gov.uk/government/publications/working-together-to-safeguard-children–2

Department of Health and Social Care (DHSC) (2021a) *NHS Mandate 2021 to 2022 Policy Paper.* Available at: https://www.gov.uk/government/publications/nhs-mandate-2021-to-2022

Department of Health and Social Care (DHSC) (2021b) *Transforming the Public Health System: Reforming the Public Health System for the Challenges of Our Times.* Available at: https://www.gov.uk/government/publications/transforming-the-public-health-system

Department of Health and Social Care (DHSC) (2021c) *Integration and Innovation: Working Together to Improve Health and Social Care for All.* Available at: https://www.gov.uk/government/publications/working-together-to-improve-health-and-social-care-for-all

Department of Health and Social Security (DHSS) (1986) *Neighbourhood Nursing: A Focus for Care* (Cumberlege report). London: HMSO.

Department of Health and Social Security (DHSS) (1992) Medicinal Products; Prescriptions by Nurses etc. *Act.* London: HMSO.

Diabetes UK (2019) *Reversing Type 2 Diabetes* [online]. Available at: https://www.diabetes.co.uk/reversing-diabetes.html

Diamond-Fox, S (2021) Understanding consultations and clinical assessments at advanced level. *British Journal of Nursing, 30*(4): 238–43.

DiCenso, A, Cullum, N and Ciliska, D (1998) Implementing evidence-based nursing: some misconceptions. *Evidence-based Nursing, 1*(1): 38–9.

DiCenso, A, Bayley, L and Haynes, RB (2009) Accessing pre-appraised evidence: fine-tuning the 5S model into a 6S model. *Evidence-Based Nursing, 12*: 99–101. Available at: https://ebn.bmj.com/content/12/4/99.2

Dickson, CAW and Peelo-Kilroe, L (2021) Being person-centred in community and ambulatory contexts, in McCormack, B, McCance, T, Brown, D, Bulley, C, McMillan, A and Martin, S (eds) *Becoming a Person-centred Health Care Practitioner: Flourishing Through Learning.* London: Blackwell.

Djerbib, A (2018) A qualitative systematic review of the factors that influence prescribing decisions by nurse independent prescribers in primary care. *Primary Healthcare, 28*(3): 25–34.

Dossey, B and Guzetta, C (2015) *Holistic Nursing: A Handbook for Practice* (4th edn). Boston: Jones and Bartlett.

Drennan, VM, Grant, RL and Harris, R (2014) Trends over time in prescribing by English primary care nurses: a secondary analysis of a national prescription database. *BMC Health Services Research, 14*(54). Available at: https://doi.org/10.1186/1472-6963-14-54

Drinkwater, C, Wildman, J and Moffatt, S (2019) Social prescribing. *British Medical Journal, 364.* Available at: https://www.bmj.com/content/364/bmj.l1285

Duncan, D and Johnstone, J (2018) Prescriber ready – are you ready? *Nurse Prescribing, 16*(7): 345–7.

Eccleston, C (2019) The multi-disciplinary prescribing team, in Nuttall, D and Rutt-Howard, J (eds) *The Textbook of Non-Medical Prescribing.* Newark, NJ: John Wiley & Sons.

Electronic Medicines Compendium (eMC) Available at: www.medicines.org.uk

Electronic Medicines Compendium (eMC) Medicines.org (2017) *Warfarin Tablets: Summary of product characteristics.* Available at: https://www.medicines.org.uk/emc/product/3064/smpc

Electronic Medicines Compendium (eMC) Medicines.org (2019) *Diazepam Tablets 5 mg: Summary of product characteristics.* Available at: https://www.medicines.org.uk/emc/product/4524/smpc#gref

Electronic Medicines Compendium (eMC) Medicines.org (2020a) *Anadin Paracetamol Tablets: Summary of product characteristics.* Available at: https://www.medicines.org.uk/emc/product/11899/smpc

Electronic Medicines Compendium (eMC) Medicines.org (2020b) *Paracetamol 10 mg/ml Solution for Infusion: Summary of product characteristics.* Available at: https://www.medicines.org.uk/emc/product/2972/smpc

Electronic Medicines Compendium (eMC) Medicines.org (2021a) *Amitriptyline SPC: Summary of product characteristics.* Available at: https://www.medicines.org.uk/emc/product/5698/smpc

Electronic Medicines Compendium (eMC) Medicines.org (2021b) *Cisplatin: Summary of product characteristics.* https://www.medicines.org.uk/emc/medicine/623#gref

Electronic Medicines Compendium (eMC) Medicines.org (2021c) *Orkambi: Summary of product characteristics.* Available at: https://www.medicines.org.uk/emc/product/9845/smpc

Elliott, R, Camacho, E, Campbell, F, Jankovic, D, *et al.* (2018) *Prevalence and Economic Burden of Medication Errors in the NHS in England: Rapid Evidence Synthesis and Economic Analysis of the Prevalence and Burden of Medication Error in the UK. Policy Research Unit in Economic Evaluation of Health and Care Interventions. Universities of Sheffield and York [online].* Available at: http://www.eepru.org.uk/prevalence-and-economic-burden-of-medication-errors-in-the-nhs-in-england-2/

Embleton, R and Henderson, M (2020) Overcoming barriers to nurses performing digital rectal examination. *Nursing Times* [online], *116*(9): 42–4.

Emrich-Mills, L, Collier, P and West, J (2019) The role of nurse prescribers in memory services and their continuing professional development: a review of the literature. *Journal of Clinical Nursing, 28*: 1422–32. Available at: https://doi.org/10.1111/jocn.14796

European Medicines Agency (2014) *Good Practice Guide on Risk Minimisation and Prevention of Medication Errors* EMA/606103/2014. Available at: https://www.ema.europa.eu/en/human-regulatory/post-authorisation/pharmacovigilance/medication-errors

Evidence Alerts Available at: https://www.evidencealerts.com

Faculty of Pain Medicine (FPM) (2020) *Opioids Aware* Available at: https://www.fpm.ac.uk/opioids-aware

Family Law Reform Act 1969. Available at: http://www.legislation.gov.uk/ukpga/1969/46

Family Law Reform Act 1987. Available at: https://www.legislation.gov.uk/ukpga/1987/42

Fancourt, D and Finn, S (2019) *What is the evidence on the role of the arts in improving health and wellbeing?* A scoping review. Health Evidence Network synthesis report 67. World Health Organization. Available at: http://www.euro.who.int/en/publications/abstracts/what-is-the-evidence-on-the-role-of-the-arts-in-improving-health-and-well-being-a-scoping-review-2019

Fletcher, J, Atkin, L, Dowsett, C, Gardner, S, Schofield, A, Staines, K and Vowden, K (2019) *Best Practice Statement: Addressing Complexities in the Management of Venous Leg Ulcers.* 30 April. Wounds UK. Available at: https://www.wounds-uk.com/resources/details/best-practice-statement-addressing-complexities-management-venous-leg-ulcers

Fletcher, J, Atkin, L, Dowsett, C, Hopkins, A, Tickle, J, Worboys, F and Williams, A (2016) *Best Practice Statement Best Practice Statement: Holistic management of venous leg ulceration* January 2016, Wounds UK. Available at: https://www.wounds-uk.com/resources/details/best-practice-statement-holistic-management-of-venous-leg-ulceration

Ford, K and Otway, C (2008) Health visitor prescribing: the need for CPD. *Nurse Prescribing*, 6(9): 387–403.

Francis, R (Mid Staffordshire NHS Foundation Trust Public Inquiry) (2013) *Report of the Mid Staffordshire NHS Foundation Trust Public Inquiry: Executive Summary.* Available at: https://www.gov.uk/government/publications/report-of-the-mid-staffordshire-nhs-foundation-trust-public-inquiry

Franklin, P (2006) Non-medical prescribing and the community practitioner; fit for purpose? *Community Practitioner*, 79(12): 388–9.

Freeman, J (2005) Towards a definition of holism. *British Journal of General Practice*, February: 154–5.

General Medical Council (GMC) (2018a) *Consent: Patients and Doctors Making Decisions Together.* Available at: https://www.gmc-uk.org/guidance/ethical_guidance/consent_guidance_index.asp

General Medical Council (GMC) (2018b) *0–18 Guidance for All Doctors.* Available at: https://www.gmc-uk.org/ethical-guidance/ethical-guidance-for-doctors/0-18-years

General Medical Council (GMC) (2021) *Good Practice in Prescribing and Managing Medicines and Devices: Prescribing Unlicensed Medicines* [online]. Available at: https://www.gmc-uk.org/ethical-guidance/ethical-guidance-for-doctors/good-practice-in-prescribing-and-managing-medicines-and-devices

Georgieva, JV, Hoekstra, D and Zuhorn, IS (2014) Smuggling drugs into the brain: an overview of ligands targeting transcytosis for drug delivery across the blood–brain barrier. *Pharmaceutics*, 6(4): 557–83. Available at: https://doi.org/10.3390/pharmaceutics6040557

Gillick v West Norfolk and Wisbech AHA AC 112 ((HL)) 1986. Available at: http://www.hrcr.org/safrica/childrens_rights/Gillick_WestNorfolk.htm

Gough, H (2018) Community nursing assessment in Chiltern S and Bain H (editors) (2018) *A textbook of community nursing* (2nd edn). London: Routledge

Gounden, V, Vashisht, R and Jialal, I (2020) Hypoalbuminemia, in *StatPearls* [online]. Treasure Island, FL: StatPearls. Available at: https://www.ncbi.nlm.nih.gov/books/NBK526080/

Green, J, Jester, R, McKinley, R, Pooler, A, Mason, S and Redsell, S (2015) A new quality of life consultation template for patients with venous leg ulceration. *Journal of Wound Care, 24*(1).

Green, J, Corcoran, P, Green, L and Read, S (2018a) A new quality of life wound checklist: the patient voice in wound care. *Wounds UK, 14*(4): 40–5.

Green, J, Jester, R, McKinley, R and Pooler, A (2018b) Chronic venous leg ulcer care: putting the patient at the heart of leg ulcer care. Part 1: exploring the consultation. *British Journal of Community Nursing, 23*(Sup3): S30–S38.

Griffith, R (2008) Consent and children: the law for children under sixteen. *British Journal of School Nursing, 3*(6).

Griffith, R (2012) Medicines law overhaul with Human Medicines Regulations. *British Journal of School Nursing, 17*(9): 445–7. Available at: https://doi.org/10.12968/bjcn.2012.17.9.445

Griffith, R (2013) Nurses must be more confident in assessing Gillick competence. *British Journal of Nursing, 22*(12).

Griffith, R (2015) Understanding the Code: use of medicines. *British Journal of Community Nursing, 20*(12).

Griffith, R (2018) Neglect by carers. *British Journal of Community Nursing, 23*(8).

Griffith, R (2019) Negligence and the standard of care in district nursing. *British Journal of Community Nursing, 24*(1).

Griffith, R and Tengnah, C (2011) Legal issues surrounding consent and capacity: the key to autonomy. *British Journal of Community Nursing, 16*(12). Available at: https://www.ncbi.nlm.nih.gov/pubmed/22413407

Griffith, R and Tengnah, C (2012) Consent to care: patients who demand or refuse treatment. *Journal of Community Nursing, 17*(3). Available at: https://www.ncbi.nlm.nih.gov/pubmed/22398872

Griffith, R and Tengnah, C (2017) *Law and Professional Issues in Nursing (Transforming Nursing Practice Series)* (4th edn). London: Sage.

Guest, JF, Fuller, GW and Vowden, P (2018) Diabetic foot ulcer management in clinical practice in the UK: costs and outcomes. *International Wound Journal, 15*: 43–52. Available at: https://onlinelibrary.wiley.com/doi/full/10.1111/iwj.12816

Guest, JF, Fuller, GW and Vowden, P (2020) Cohort study evaluating the burden of wounds to the UK's National Health Service in 2017/2018: update from 2012/2013. *BMJ Open; 10*:e045253. Available at: https://bmjopen.bmj.com/content/10/12/e045253

Gunowa, N, Hutchinson, M, Brooke, J and Jackson, D (2018) Pressure injuries in people with darker skin tones: a literature review. *Journal of Clinical Nursing*, 27(17–18): 3266–75. Available at: https://pubmed.ncbi.nlm.nih.gov/28887872/

Hall, K and Picton, C (2020) Analysing the Competency Framework for All Prescribers. *Journal of Prescribing Practice*, 2(3): 122–8.

Ham, C, Alderwick, H, Dunn, P and McKenna, H (2017) Delivering sustainability and transformation plans: from ambitious proposals to credible plans [online]. Available at: https://www.kingsfund.org.uk/publications/delivering-sustainability-and-transformation-plans

Hampton, J, Harrison, M, Mitchell, R, Prichard, S and Seymour, C (1975) Relative contributions of history-taking, physical examination, and laboratory investigation to diagnosis and management of medical outpatients. *British Medical Journal*, 2(5969): 486–9.

Harper, C and Ajao, A (2013) Pendleton's consultation model: assessing a patient. *British Journal of Community Nursing*, 15(1). Available at: https://doi.org/10.12968/bjcn.2010.15.1.45784

Hastings, A and Redsall, S (2006a) *The Good Consultation Guide for Nurses*. Abingdon: Radcliffe.

Hastings A. and Redsall S. (2006b) Using the Consultation Assessment and Improvement Instrument for Nurses (CAIIN) in Assessment [online]. Available at: https://www.researchgate.net/publication/254757754_Using_the_Consultation_Assessment_and_Improvement_Instrument_for_Nurses_CAIIN_in_assessment

Hawkley, L, Thisted, R, Masi, C and Cacioppo, JT (2010) Loneliness predicts increased blood pressure: 5-year cross-lagged analyses in middle-aged and older adults. *Psychology and Aging*, 25(1): 132–41. doi: 10.1037/a0017805

Health and Social Care Act (2015). Available at: https://navigator.health.org.uk/theme/health-and-social-care-safety-and-quality-act-2015

Health Protection Surveillance Centre (2021) Notifiable diseases. Available at: https://www.hpsc.ie/notifiablediseases/

Health Safety Investigation Branch (HSIB) (2021a) *Unintentional overdose of paracetamol in adults with low bodyweight*. Available at: https://www.hsib.org.uk/investigations-cases/unintentional-overdose-paracetamol-adults-low-bodyweight/

Health Safety Investigation Branch (HSIB) (2021b) *Weight-based medication errors in children*. Available at: https://www.hsib.org.uk/investigations-cases/weight-based-medication-errors-children/

Hewitt-Taylor, J (2006) *Clinical Guidelines and Care Protocols*. Bournemouth: Wiley & Sons.

Holmes, K (2006) Maintaining prescribing standards should silence the critics. *Nurse Prescribing*, 4: 413–15.

Holt-Lunstad, J, Smith, T, Baker, M, Harris, T and Stephenson, D (2015) Loneliness and social isolation as risk factors for mortality: a meta-analytic review. *Perspectives on Psychological Science*, 10(2): 227–37.

Howick, J, Chalmers, I, Glasziou, P, Greenhalgh, T, *et al.* (2011) *The 2011 Oxford CEBM Evidence Levels of Evidence (Introductory Document).* Oxford Centre for Evidence-Based Medicine. Available at: http://www.cebm.net/index.aspx?o=5653

Human Medicines Regulations (2012). Available at: https://www.legislation.gov.uk/uksi/2012/1916/contents/made

i5 Health (2015) *Non-medical Prescribing: An Economic Evaluation.* Health Education North West. Available at: http://www.i5health.com/NMP/NMPEconomicEvaluation.pdf

International Union of Basic and Clinical Pharmacology (IUPHAR) (2021) *Ion Channels (Ligand-gated Ion Channels).* Available at: https://www.pharmacologyeducation.org/pharmacology/ion-channels

Joint Formulary Committee (JFC) *British National Formulary* [online]. London: BMJ Group and Pharmaceutical Press. Available at: https://bnf.nice.org.uk

Kennedy, CM (2004) A typology of knowledge for district nursing. *Journal of Advanced Nursing, 45*(4): 401–9.

Kennedy, I and Grubb, A (1998) *Principles of Medical Law.* Oxford: Oxford University Press.

Kennedy, I (2001) *Bristol Royal Infirmary Inquiry: The Report of the Public Inquiry into children's heart surgery at the Bristol Royal Infirmary 1984–1995 Learning from Bristol.* Available at: https://webarchive.nationalarchives.gov.uk/20090811143822/http:/www.bristol-inquiry.org.uk/final_report/the_report.pdf

Keers, R, Williams, S, Vattakatuchery, J, Brown, P, Miller, J and Prescott, L (2015) Medication safety at the interface: evaluating risks associated with discharge prescriptions from mental health hospitals. *Journal of Clinical Pharmacy and Therapeutics, 40*(6): 645–54.

Klein, J, Delany, C and Fischer, MD (2017) A growth mindset approach to preparing trainees for medical error. *British Medical Journal Quality and Safety, 26*: 771–4.

Kurtz, SM, Silverman, JD and Draper J (1998) *Teaching and Learning Communication Skills in Medicine.* Oxford: Radcliffe Medical Press.

Latter, S and Courtenay, M (2004) Effectiveness of nurse prescribing: a review of the literature. *Journal of Clinical Nursing, 13*(1): 26–32.

Latter, S, Maben, J, Myall, M, Courtenay, M, *et al.* (2005a) *Evaluation of Extended Formulary Independent Nurse Prescribing: Executive Summary of Final Report* (Policy Research Programme – Department of Health and University of Southampton). Available at: http://eprints.soton.ac.uk/17584/

Latter, S, Maben, J, Myall, M, Courtenay, M, *et al.* (2005b) *Evaluation of Extended Formulary Independent Nurse Prescribing: Final Report* (Policy Research Programme – Department of Health and University of Southampton).

Latter, S, Maben, J, Myall, M and Young, A (2007) Evaluating nurse prescribers' education and continuing professional development for independent prescribing practice: findings from a national survey in England. *Nurse Education Today, 27*: 685–96.

Latter, S, Blenkinsopp, A, Smith, A, Chapman, S, *et al.* (2010) *Evaluation of Nurse and Pharmacist Independent Prescribing: Department of Health Policy Research Programme Project 016 0108.* Available at: http://eprints.soton.ac.uk/184777/3/ENPIPfullreport.pdf

Latter, S, Blenkinsopp, A, Smith, A, Chapman, S, *et al.* (2011) *Evaluation of Nurse and Pharmacist Independent Prescribing.* Department of Health England: http://eprints.soton. ac.uk/184777/2/ENPIPexecsummary.pdf

Lencioni, P (2002) *The Five Dysfunctions of a Team.* San Francisco: Jossey-Bass.

Lim, AG, North, N and Shaw, J (2018) Beginners in prescribing practice: experiences and perceptions of nurses and doctors. *Journal of Clinical Nursing, 27*: 1103–12. Available at: https://doi.org/10.1111/jocn.14136

Luker, B, Austin, l, Hogg, B, Ferguson, B, *et al.* (1997) Nurse prescribing: the views of nurses and other health care professionals. *British Journal of Community Health Nursing, 2*(2): 69–74.

Luker, B, Austin, l, Hogg, B, Ferguson, B, *et al.* (1998) Nurse–patient relationships: the context of nurse prescribing. *Journal of Advanced Nursing, 28*(2): 235–42.

Luo, Y, Hawkley, L, Waite, L and Cacippio, J (2012) Loneliness, health and mortality in old age: a longitudinal study. *Social Science and Medicine, 74*(6): 907–14.

Lynas, K (2013) Introduction to Team Development NHS Leadership Academy [online]. Available at: https://www.leadershipacademy.nhs.uk/wp-content/uploads/20 13/04/7428f23d7207f39da1eda97adbd7bf34.pdf

Maben, J, Peccei, R, Adams, M, Robert, G, Richardson, A, Murrells, T and Morrow, E (2012) *Exploring the Relationship between Patients' Experiences of Care and the Influence of Staff Motivation, Affect and Wellbeing.* London: National Institute for Health Research Service Delivery and Organisation Programme.

Magowan, J (2020) Barriers and enablers to nurse prescribing in primary care. *Journal of Prescribing Practice, 2*(3): 142–6.

Marmot, M, Allen, J, Boyce, T, Goldblatt, P and McNeish, D (2010) *Fair Society, Healthy Lives (The Marmot Review)* [online]. Available at: https://www.instituteofhealthequity. org/resources-reports/fair-society-healthy-lives-the-marmot-review

Marmot, M, Allen, J, Boyce, T, Goldblatt, P and Morrison, J (2020) *Health Equity in England: The Marmot Review 10 Years On* [online]. Available at: https://www.health.org. uk/publications/reports/the-marmot-review-10-years-on

Maybin, J, Charles, A and Honeyman, H (2016) *Understanding Quality in District Nursing Services: Learning from Patients, Carers and Staff.* London: The King's Fund. Available at: www.kingsfund.org.uk/publications/quality-district-nursing

McCance, T, McCormack, B, Brown, D, Bulley, C, McMillan, A and Martin, S (2021) *Fundamentals of Person-Centred Healthcare Practice.* Oxford: Wiley Global Research (STMS). Available at: VitalSource Bookshelf

McDonald, A (2016) *The Long and Winding Road: Improving Communication with Patients in the NHS* [ebook]: 18. London: Marie Curie. Available at: https://www.mariecurie.org. uk/globalassets/media/documents/policy/campaigns/the-long-and-winding-road.pdf

McHugh, Á, Hughes, M, Higgins, A, Buckley, T, *et al.* (2020) Non-medical prescribers: prescribing within practice. *Journal of Prescribing Practice,* 2(2): 68–77.

McIntosh, T, Stewart, D, Forbes-McKay, K, McCaig, D and Cunningham, S (2016) Influences on prescribing decision-making among non-medical prescribers in the United Kingdom: systematic review. *Family Practice,* 33(6): 572–9.

McKenna, B (2020) Impact of COVID-19 on prescribing in English general practice: March 2020 [online]. 20 May. Available at: https://ebmdatalab.net/covid19-prescribing-impact/

Medicines Act [1968]. Available at: https://www.legislation.gov.uk/ukpga/1968/67

Medicines and Healthcare Products Regulatory Agency (MHRA) (2005) *Consultation on Options for the Future of Independent Prescribing by Extended Formulary Nurse Prescribers.* London: DoH. Gateway Reference 4437

Medicines and Healthcare Products Regulatory Agency (MHRA) (2006) *Summary of Replies to the Consultation on Options for the Future of Independent Prescribing by Extended Formulary Nurse Prescribers.* London: DoH.

Medicines and Healthcare Products Regulatory Agency (MHRA) (2014) *Rules for the Sale, Supply and Administration of Medicines for Specific Healthcare Professionals* [online]. Available at: https://www.gov.uk/government/publications/rules-for-the-sale-supply-and-administration-of-medicines/rules-for-the-sale-supply-and-administration-of-medicines-for-specific-healthcare-professionals

Medicines and Healthcare Products Regulatory Agency (MHRA) (2015) *Guidance on Adverse Drug Reaction.* Available at: http://www.mhra.gov.uk. Link to PDF https://assets.publishing.service.gov.uk/government/uploads/system/uploads/attachment_data/file/949130/Guidance_on_adverse_drug_reactions.pdf

Medicines and Healthcare Products Regulatory Agency (MHRA) (2017) *Patient Group Directions (PGDs): Who Can Use Them?* Available at: https://www.gov.uk/government/publications/patient-group-directions-pgds/patient-group-directions-who-can-use-them

Medicines and Healthcare Products Regulatory Agency (MHRA) (2019) *The Yellow Card Scheme: Guidance for Healthcare Professionals.* Available at: www.mhra.gov.uk

Medicines and Healthcare Products Regulatory Agency (MHRA) (2020) *Opioids: Risk of Dependence and Addiction.* Available at: https://www.gov.uk/drug-safety-update/opioids-risk-of-dependence-and-addiction

Medicines for Human Use (Prescribing) (Miscellaneous Amendments) Order [2006]. Available at: https://www.legislation.gov.uk/uksi/2006/915/contents/made?view=plain

Medicinal Products: Prescription by Nurses etc. Act 1992 (c. 28). Available at: https://www.legislation.gov.uk/ukpga/1992/28/contents

Medicines Optimisation Resources. Available at: https://www.england.nhs.uk/medicines-2/medicines-optimisation/

MedlinePlus (2020a) Medical encyclopedia: *Intestinal obstruction.* Available at: https://medlineplus.gov/intestinalobstruction.html

MedlinePlus (2020b) Medical encyclopedia: *Gastrointestinal perforation.* Available at: https://medlineplus.gov/ency/article/000235.htm

Mehrabian, A (1972) *Nonverbal Communication.* New Brunswick: Aldine Transaction.

Mental Capacity Act [2005] Available at: http://www.legislation.gov.uk/ukpga/2005/9/contents

Mental Health Act [1983] Available at: https://www.legislation.gov.uk/ukpga/1983/20/contents

Misuse of Drugs Act [1971] Available at: https://www.legislation.gov.uk/ukpga/1971/38/contents

Misuse of Drugs Act Amendment number 2 [2012]. Available at: https://www.legislation.gov.uk/nisr/2012/213/contents/made

Misuse of Drugs regulations [2001]. Available at: https://www.legislation.gov.uk/uksi/2001/3998/contents/made

Moman, RN, Gupta, N and Varacallo, M (2020) Physiology, Albumin. 22 September, in *StatPearls* [online]. Treasure Island (FL): StatPearls. Available at: https://www.ncbi.nlm.nih.gov/books/NBK459198/

Montgomery v Lanarkshire Health Board [2015] Available at: https://www.supremecourt.uk/cases/uksc-2013-0136.html

Mukwende, M, Tamony, P and Turner, M (2020) *Mind the Gap: A Handbook of Clinical Signs in Black and Brown Skin.* St George's, University of London. Available at: https://doi.org/10.24376/rd.sgul.12769988.v1

Muncey, R (2018) The impact of health visitor prescribing and advice on parent/carer use of GP services. *Journal of Health Visiting,* 6(11): 562–6.

Mundinger, M, Kane, R, Lenz, E, Totten A *et al.* (2000) Primary care outcomes in patients treated by nurse practitioners or physicians: a randomised control trial. *Journal of American Medical Association, 283*: 59–68.

Munroe, B, Curtis, K, Considine, J, *et al.* (2013) The impact structured patient assessment frameworks have on patient care: an integrative review, in Database of Abstracts of Reviews of Effects (DARE): Quality-assessed Reviews [online]. York: Centre for Reviews and Dissemination. Available at: https://www.ncbi.nlm.nih.gov/books/NBK138388

Murad, M, Asi, N, Alsawas, M, *et al.* (2016) New evidence pyramid. *BMJ Evidence-Based Medicine, 21*: 125–7.

Naito, T, Tashiro, M, Yamamoto, K *et al.* (2012) Impact of cachexia on pharmacokinetic disposition of and clinical responses to oxycodone in cancer patients. *European Journal of Clinical Pharmacology, 68*: 1411–18. Available at: https://doi.org/10.1007/s00228-012-1266-x

National Health Service Act 1977. Available at: https://www.legislation.gov.uk/ukpga/1977/49/contents

National Health Service (NHS) (2019) *The NHS Long Term Plan.* Available at: https://www.longtermplan.nhs.uk/

NHSBSA Catalyst. Available at: https://www.england.nhs.uk/medicines-2/medicines-optimisation/ and https://managemeds.scot.nhs.uk

NHS Digital (2019a) *Electronic Prescription Services* [online]. Available at: https://digital.nhs.uk/services/electronic-prescription-service

NHS Digital (2019b) *The National Diabetes Foot Care Audit (NDFA).* Available at: https://digital.nhs.uk/data-and-information/publications/statistical/national-diabetes-footcare-audit/2014-2018

NHS Digital (2020) *Prescribing Costs in Hospitals and the Community.* Available at: https://digital.nhs.uk/data-and-information/publications/statistical/prescribing-costs-in-hospitals-and-the-community

NHS England (2014) *Improving Medication Error Incident Reporting and Learning: Patient Safety Alert Directive.* NHS/PSA/D/2014/005. Available at: https://www.england.nhs.uk/wp-content/uploads/2014/03/psa-sup-info-med-error.pdf

NHS England (2019) *National Patient Safety Alerts.* Available at: https://www.england.nhs.uk/patient-safety/national-patient-safety-alerting-committee/

NHS England (2020) *Patient Safety Incident Management System.* Available at: https://www.england.nhs.uk/patient-safety/patient-safety-incident-management-system/

NHS England (2021a) *The Medicine Safety Improvement Programme.* Available at: https://www.england.nhs.uk/patient-safety/national-medicines-safety-programme/

NHS England (2021b) NHS 111 Minimum Data Set 2020–21 [online]. Available at: https://www.england.nhs.uk/statistics/statistical-work-areas/nhs-111-minimum-data-set/nhs-111-minimum-data-set-2020-21/

NHS England and NHS Improvement (2017) *Active Listening* [online]. Available at: https://www.england.nhs.uk/quality-service-improvement-and-redesign-qsir-tools/

NHS Improvement (2016) *National Reporting and Learning System Data Principles* [online]. Available at: https://improvement.nhs.uk/resources/learning-from-patient-safety-incidents/#h2-how-nrls-data-should-be-used

NHS Improvement (2018a) *Learning from Patient Safety Incidents.* Available at: https://webarchive.nationalarchives.gov.uk/ukgwa/20200706210038/https:/improvement.nhs.uk/resources/learning-from-patient-safety-incidents/

NHS Improvement (2018b) *Patient Safety Alert: Resources to Support Safer Bowel Care for Patients at Risk of Autonomic Dysreflexia.* Available at: https://www.england.nhs.uk/2018/07/patients-at-risk-of-autonomic-dysreflexia/

NHS Scotland (2014) Scottish Management of Antimicrobial Resistance Action Plan 2014–18 (ScotMARAP2). Available at: https://www.gov.scot/publications/scottish-management-antimicrobial-resistance-action-plan-2014-18-scotmarap2/

National Institute of Health and Care Excellence (NICE) evidence. Available at: https://www.evidence.nhs.uk

National Institute of Health and Care Excellence (NICE) Available at: https://www.nice.org.uk/about/nice-communities/medicines-and-prescribing

References

National Institute for Health and Care Excellence (2008) *Social Value Judgements: Principles for the Development of NICE Guidance,* Version 2. 31 July. Available: https://www.nice.org.uk/about/who-we-are/our-principles

National Institute of Health and Care Excellence (NICE) (2015a) *Pressure Ulcers Quality Standard [QS89]* [online]. Available at: https://www.nice.org.uk/guidance/qs89/chapter/Quality-statement-4-Skin-assessment

National Institute of Health and Care Excellence (NICE) (2015b) *Antimicrobial Stewardship: Systems and Processes for Effective Antimicrobial Medicines Use.* London: NICE [NICE guidelines NG15]. Available at: https://www.nice.org.uk/guidance/ng15/resources/antimicrobial-stewardship-systemsand-processes-for-effective-antimicrobial-medicine-use-pdf-1837273110469

National Institute of Health and Care Excellence (NICE) (2015c) *Naloxegol for Treating Opioid-induced Constipation: Technology Appraisal Guidance [TA345].* Available at: https://www.nice.org.uk/guidance/ta345

National Institute of Health and Care Excellence (NICE) (2016a) Antimicrobial Stewardship Quality Standard [QS121] [online]. Available at: https://www.nice.org.uk/guidance/qs121

National Institute for Health and Care Excellence (2016b) Chronic Wounds: Advanced Wound Dressings and Antimicrobial Dressings: Evidence Summary [ESMPB2] [online]. Available at: https://www.nice.org.uk/advice/esmpb2/chapter/Full-evidence-summary-medicines-and-prescribing-briefing

National Institute of Health and Care Excellence (NICE) (2017a) *Patient Group Directives.* Available at: https://www.nice.org.uk/guidance/mpg2/chapter/recommendations#considering-the-need-for-a-patient-group-direction

National Institute for Health and Care Excellence (2017b) *Antimicrobial Stewardship: Changing Risk-related Behaviours in the General Population NICE Guideline [NG63].* Available at: https://www.nice.org.uk/guidance/ng63

National Institute for Health and Care Excellence (2017c) *Suspected Cancer: Recognition and Referral.* Available at: https://www.nice.org.uk/guidance/ng12

National Institute of Health and Care Excellence (NICE) (2018a) *Decision-making and Mental Capacity NICE Guideline [NG108]* [online]. Available at: https://www.nice.org.uk/guidance/ng108

National Institute for Health and Care Excellence (2018b) *Promoting Health and Preventing Premature Mortality in Black, Asian and Other Minority Ethnic Groups Quality Standard [QS167].* Available at: https://www.nice.org.uk/guidance/qs167

National Institute of Health and Care Excellence (NICE) (2018c) Clinical Knowledge Summaries (CKS). *Adverse Drug Reactions.* Available at: https://cks.nice.org.uk/adverse-drug-reactions#!scenario

National Institute of Health and Care Excellence (NICE) (2018d) Clinical Knowledge Summaries (CKS). *Head Lice* [online]. Available at: https://cks.nice.org.uk/head-lice

National Institute of Health and Care Excellence (NICE) (2019a) *Diabetic Foot Problems: Prevention and Management* NICE guideline [NG19] [online]. Available at: https://www.nice.org.uk/guidance/ng19

National Institute for Health and Care Excellence (2019b) *Consensus Based National Antimicrobial Stewardship Competencies for UK Undergraduate Healthcare Professional Education.* Available at: https://www.nice.org.uk/sharedlearning/consensus-based-national-antimicrobial-stewardship-competencies-for-uk-undergraduate-healthcare-professional-education

National Institute of Health and Care Excellence (NICE) (2020a) Developing NICE Guidelines: The Manual (PMG20) Appendix H Appraisal checklists, evidence tables, GRADE and economic profiles. Available at: https://www.nice.org.uk/process/pmg20/resources/appendix-h-appraisal-checklistsevidence-tables-grade-and-economic-profiles-pdf-8779777885

National Institute of Health and Care Excellence (NICE) (2020b) *Naldemedine for Treating Opioid-induced Constipation: Technology Appraisal Guidance [TA651].* Available at: https://www.nice.org.uk/guidance/ta651

National Institute for Health and Care Excellence (NICE) (2020c) Clinical Knowledge Summaries (CKS) *Constipation.* Available at: https://cks.nice.org.uk/topics/constipation/

National Institute for Health and Care Excellence (NICE) (2020d) Clinical Knowledge Summaries (CKS) *Constipation in Children.* Available at: https://cks.nice.org.uk/topics/constipation-in-children/

National Institute for Health and Care Excellence (NICE) (2020e) *Leg Ulcer Infection: Antimicrobial Prescribing.* NICE guideline [NG152]. Available at: https://www.nice.org.uk/guidance/ng152

National Institute for Health and Care Excellence (NICE) (2021a) *Atrial Fibrillation: Medicines to Help Reduce your Risk of a Stroke: What are the Options?* Patient decision aid. Available at: https://www.nice.org.uk/guidance/cg180/resources

National Institute for Health and Care Excellence (2021b) *Behaviour Change.* Available at: https://www.nice.org.uk/guidance/lifestyle-and-wellbeing/behaviour-change

National Institute of Health and Care Excellence (NICE) (2021c) Clinical Knowledge Summaries (CKS) *Atopic Eczema* [online]. Available at: https://cks.nice.org.uk/eczema-atopic#!scenario:1

National Institute of Health and Care Excellence (NICE) (2021d) Clinical Knowledge Summaries (CKS) *How to Assess Infected Lacerations* [online]. Available at: https://cks.nice.org.uk/topics/lacerations/diagnosis/assessment/

National Institute for Health and Care Excellence (NICE) (2021e) Clinical Knowledge Summaries (CKS) *Opioid dependence.* Available at: https://cks.nice.org.uk/topics/opioid-dependence/

National Institute for Health and Care Excellence (NICE) (2021f) Clinical Knowledge Summaries (CKS) *Mastitis and Breast Abscess.* Available at: https://cks.nice.org.uk/topics/mastitis-breast-abscess/

National Institute for Health and Care Excellence (NICE) (2021g) Clinical Knowledge Summaries (CKS) *Leg Ulcers: Venous.* Available at: https://cks.nice.org.uk/topics/leg-ulcer-venous/

National Institute for Health and Care Excellence (NICE) (2021h) Clinical Knowledge Summaries (CKS) *Gastrointestinal Tract (Lower) Cancers: Recognition and Referral.* Available at: https://cks.nice.org.uk/topics/gastrointestinal-tract-lower-cancers-recognition-referral/

National Institute of Health and Care Excellence (NICE)/Joint Formulary Committee (JFC) Available at: https://bnf.nice.org.uk

National Institute of Health and Care Excellence (NICE)/Nurse Prescribers' Advisory Group (NPAG) *Nurse Prescribers' Formulary.* Available at: https://bnf.nice.org.uk/nurse-prescribers-formulary/

National Prescribing Centre (NPC) (1999a) Signposts for prescribing nurses: general principles of good prescribing. *Nurse Prescribing Bulletin, 1*: 1–4.

National Prescribing Centre (NPC) (1999b) *The Prescribing Pyramid Fact Sheet No.3,* September.

Neighbour, R (1987) *The Inner Consultation.* Oxford: Radcliffe Medical Press.

Newton, C (1991) *The Roper-Logan-Tierney Model in Action.* Basingstoke: Macmillan.

Nigam, Y, Knight, J and Williams, N (2019) Gastrointestinal tract 5: the anatomy and functions of the large intestine. *Nursing Times* [online], *115*(10): 50–3. Available at: https://www.nursingtimes.net/clinical-archive/gastroenterology/gastrointestinal-tract-5-anatomy-functions-large-intestine-23-09-2019/

Nimmo, S, Paterson, R and Irvin, L (2017) CPD needs of opioid nurse prescribers: a survey. *Nurse Prescribing, 15*(6): 297–302. Available at: https://www.magonlinelibrary.com/doi/abs/10.12968/npre.2017.15.6.297

Noblet, T, Marriott, J, Graham-Clarke, E and Rushton, A (2017) Barriers to and facilitators of independent non-medical prescribing in clinical practice: a mixed-methods systematic review. *Journal of Physiotherapy* [online], *63*: 221–34. Available at: https://doi.org/10.1016/j.jphys.2017.09.001

Nursing and Midwifery Council (NMC) (2018a) The Code. Available at: https://www.nmc.org.uk/standards/code/

Nursing and Midwifery Council (NMC) (2018b) Future Nurse: Standards of Proficiency for Registered Nurses [online]. Available at: https://www.nmc.org.uk/standards/standards-for-nurses/standards-of-proficiency-for-registered-nurses/

Nursing and Midwifery Council (NMC) (2018c) Realising Professionalism: Standards for Education and Training Part 1: Standards Framework for Nursing and Midwifery Education [online]. Available at: https://www.nmc.org.uk/standards-for-education-and-training/standards-framework-for-nursing-and-midwifery-education/

Nursing and Midwifery Council (NMC) (2018d) Realising Professionalism: Standards for Education and Training Part 2: Standards for Student Supervision and Assessment. Available at: https://www.nmc.org.uk/globalassets/sitedocuments/education-standards/student-supervision-assessment.pdf

Nursing and Midwifery Council (NMC) (2018e) Realising Professionalism: Standards for Education and Training Part 3: Standards for Prescribing Programmes [online]. Available at: https://www.nmc.org.uk/standards/standards-for-post-registration/standards-for-prescribers/standards-for-prescribing-programmes/

Nursing and Midwifery Council (NMC) (2019a) Standards of Proficiency for Midwives [online]. Available at: https://www.nmc.org.uk/standards/standards-for-midwives/standards-of-proficiency-for-midwives/

Nursing and Midwifery Council (NMC) (2019b) High Level Principles for Good Practice in Remote Consultations and Prescribing. Available at: https://www.nmc.org.uk/standards/standards-for-post-registration/standards-for-prescribers/useful-information-for-prescribers/

Nursing and Midwifery Council (NMC) (2019c) How to Revalidate with the NMC. Available at: http://revalidation.nmc.org.uk/download-resources/guidance-and-information.html

Nursing and Midwifery Council (NMC) (2020) Annual Fitness to Practise Report 2019–2020. Available at: https://www.nmc.org.uk/about-us/reports-and-accounts/fitness-to-practise-annual-report/

Nursing and Midwifery Council (NMC) (2021) Permanent Register Data Tables (Registration data reports)

Nursing and Midwifery Order [2001] Article 19(6). Available at: https://www.legislation.gov.uk/uksi/2002/253/body/made

Open Prescribing *Prescribing Data*. Available at: https://openprescribing.net

Östman, L, Näsman, Y, Eriksson, K and Nyström, L (2019) Ethos: the heart of ethics and health. *Nursing Ethics, 26*(1): 26–36.

Ousey, K and Blackburn, J (2020) Understanding Antimicrobial Resistance and Antimicrobial Stewardship in Wound Management. Available at: https://www.wounds-uk.com/journals/issue/615/article-details/understanding-antimicrobial-resistance-and-antimicrobial-stewardship-wound-management

Øvretveit, J (1993) *Coordinating Community Care: Multidisciplinary Teams and Care Management.* Maidenhead: Open University Press.

Øvretveit, J (1997) How to describe interprofessional working, in Øvretveit, J, Matthias, P and Thompson, T (eds) *Interprofessional Working for Health and Social Care.* Community Health Series, 163–71. Basingstoke: Macmillan.

Paterson R. (2019) Continuing professional development for prescribing: what's next? *Journal of Prescribing Practice, 1*(4): 170–2.

Pendleton, D, Schofield, T, Tate, P and Havelock, P (1984) *The Consultation: An Approach to Learning and Teaching.* Oxford: Oxford University Press.

Perissinoto, C, Cenzer, I and Covinsky, K (2012) Loneliness in older persons. *Archives of Internal Medicine, 172*: 1078–84.

References

Peterson, MC, Holbrook, JH, Hales, D, Smith, NL and Staker, LV (1992) Contributions of the history, physical examination, and laboratory investigation in making medical diagnoses. *Western Journal of Medicine, 156*: 163–5.

Pharmaceutical Services Negotiating Committee (PSNC) (2019) *Dispensing and Supply: Receiving a Prescription* [online]. Available at: https://psnc.org.uk/dispensing-supply/receiving-a-prescription/is-this-prescription-form-valid/

Prendergast v Sam and Dee Ltd [1989]. Available at: https://www.i-law.com/ilaw/doc/view.htm?id=304762

Professional Standards Authority for Health and Social Care (PSA) (2020) *An Overview of Our Work and its Contribution to Protecting the Public.* Available at: https://www.professionalstandards.org.uk/publications/detail/an-overview-of-our-work-and-its-contribution-to-protecting-the-public

Professional Standards Authority for Health and Social Care (PSA) (2021a) *Performance Review: Nursing and Midwifery Council (NMC) 2019–2020.* Available at: https://www.professionalstandards.org.uk/publications/performance-review-detail/performance-review-nmc-2019-20

Professional Standards Authority for Health and Social Care (PSA) (2021b) *Professional Standards Authority Response to Regulating Healthcare Professionals, Protecting the Public.* Available at: https://www.professionalstandards.org.uk/publications/detail/professional-standards-authority-response-to-regulating-healthcare-professionals-protecting-the-public

Public Health England (PHE) (2013) *Antimicrobial Prescribing and Stewardship Competencies.* Available at: https://www.gov.uk/government/publications/antimicrobial-prescribing-and-stewardship-competencies

Public Health England (PHE) (2020) *English Surveillance Programme for Antimicrobial Utilisation and Resistance: Report 2019 to 2020.* Available at: https://www.gov.uk/government/publications/english-surveillance-programme-antimicrobial-utilisation-and-resistance-espaur-report

Public Health England (PHE) (2021) *AMR local Indicators* Available at: https://fingertips.phe.org.uk/profile/amr-local-indicators

R (Burke) v GMC [2005] EWCA 1003. Available at: https://www.bailii.org/ew/cases/EWCA/Civ/2005/1003.html

Raynor, M, Essat, Z, Ménage, D, Chapman, M and Gregory, B (2021) *The Practising Midwife, 24*(6). Available at: https://www.all4maternity.com/decolonising-midwifery-education-part-1-how-colour-aware-are-you-when-assessing-women-with-darker-skin-tones-in-midwifery-practice/

Ritter, J and Rang, HP (2019) *Rang and Dale's Pharmacology* (9th edn). Edinburgh: Elsevier.

Roper, N *et al.* (2000) *The Roper Logan and Tierney Model of Nursing.* Edinburgh: Churchill Livingstone.

Rotter, J (1954) *Social Learning and Clinical Psychology.* New York: Prentice-Hall.

Royal College of General Practitioners (RCGP) (2019) *Top Ten Tips: Dependence Forming Medications.* Available at: https://www.rcgp.org.uk/-/media/Files/CIRC/Desktop-guides/Top-Ten-Tips-Dependence-Forming-Medications-April-2019.ashx?la=en

Royal College of Nursing (RCN) (2003) *Defining Nursing.* London: RCN.

Royal College of Nursing (RCN) (2016) *The Value and Contribution of Nursing to Public Health in the UK: Final Report* [online]. London: RCN. Available at: https://www.rcn.org.uk/clinical-topics/public-health/the-role-of-nursing-staff-in-public-health

Royal College of Nursing (RCN) (2019a) *Patient Specific Directions (PSDs) and Patient Group Directions (PGDs).* Available at: https://www.rcn.org.uk/clinical-topics/medicines-management/patient-specific-directions-and-patient-group-directions

Royal College of Nursing (2019b) *Bowel Care; Management of Lower Bowel Dysfunction, including Digital Rectal Examination and Digital Removal of Faeces.* Available at: https://www.rcn.org.uk/professional-development/publications/pub-007522

Royal College of Nursing (2020a) *Prescribing Safely Under COVID-19.* Available at: https://www.rcn.org.uk/clinical-topics/medicines-management/covid-19-remote-prescribing

Royal College of Nursing (RCN) (2020b) *The Role of Nursing Staff in Public Health* [online]. London: RCN. Available at: https://www.rcn.org.uk/clinical-topics/public-health

Royal College of Nursing (2021a) *Prescribing in Pregnancy* [online]. Available at: https://www.rcn.org.uk/clinical-topics/medicines-management/prescribing-in-pregnancy

Royal College of Nursing (RCN) (2021b) *Health Protection* [online]. Available at: https://www.rcn.org.uk/clinical-topics/public-health/health-protection

Royal College of Nursing (RCN) (no date) *Medicines Management.* Available at: https://www.rcn.org.uk/clinical-topics/medicines-management

Royal Pharmaceutical Society (RPS) (2019) A Competency Framework for Designated Prescribing Practitioners. Available at: https://www.rpharms.com/resources/frameworks/designated-prescribing-practitioner-competency-framework

Royal Pharmaceutical Society (RPS) (2021a) Competency Framework for All Prescribers. Available at: https://www.rpharms.com/resources/frameworks/prescribers-competency-framework

Royal Pharmaceutical Society (RPS) (2021b) Medicines Optimisation Hub. Available at: https://www.rpharms.com/resources/pharmacy-guides/medicines-optimisation-hub

Sackett, DL, Richardson, WS, Rosenberg, W, *et al.* (2000) *Evidence-based Medicine: How to Practice and Teach EBM.* Edinburgh: Churchill Livingstone.

Samanta, A and Samanta, J (2003) Legal standard of care: a shift from the traditional Bolam test. *Clinical Medicine, 3*: 443–6. Available at: https://www.ncbi.nlm.nih.gov/pmc/articles/PMC4953641/

Scally, G and Donaldson, LJ (1998) Clinical governance and the drive for quality improvement in the new NHS in England. *British Medical Journal, 317*: 61. Available at: https://doi.org/10.1136/bmj.317.7150.61

Scottish Government (2016) *A National Clinical Strategy for Scotland* [online]. Edinburgh: Scottish Government. Available at: https://www.gov.scot/publications/national-clinical-strategy-scotland/

Scottish Government (2017) *Nursing 2030 Vision* [online]. Edinburgh, Scottish Government. Available at: https://www.gov.scot/Resource/0052/00522376.pdf

Scottish Intercollegiate Guidance Network (SIGN) (2011) *Management of Atopic Eczema in Primary Care.* Available at: https://www.sign.ac.uk/sign-125-management-of-atopic-eczema-in-primary-care.html

Scottish Intercollegiate Guidance Network (SIGN) (2017) *Management of Diabetes.* Available at: https://www.sign.ac.uk/our-guidelines/management-of-diabetes/

Scottish Intercollegiate Guidance Network (SIGN) (2019) *SIGN 50: A Guideline Developer's Handbook: SIGN Grading System 1999–2012.* Available at: https://www.sign.ac.uk/our-guidelines/sign-50-a-guideline-developers-handbook/

Scrafton, J, McKinnon, J and Kane, R (2012) Exploring nurses' experiences of prescribing in secondary care: informing future education and practice. *Journal of Clinical Nursing, 21*: 2044–53. Available at: https://doi.org/10.1111/j.1365-2702.2011.04050.x

Sharma, C and Mehta, V (2014) Paracetamol: mechanisms and updates. *Continuing Education in Anaesthesia Critical Care and Pain, 14*(4): 153–8. Available at: https://doi.org/10.1093/bjaceaccp/mkt049

Sidaway v Bethlem Royal Hospital [1985]. Available at: https://www.bailii.org/uk/cases/UKHL/1985/1.html

Silverman, JD, Kurtz, SM and Draper, J (1998) *Skills for Communicating with Patients.* Oxford: Radcliffe Medical Press.

Smith, A, Latter, S and Blenkinsopp, A (2014) Safety and quality of nurse independent prescribing: a national study of experiences of education, continuing professional development clinical governance. *Journal of Advanced Nursing, 70*(11): 2506–17. Available at: https://doi.org/10.1111/jan.12392

Soto, SM (2013) Role of efflux pumps in the antibiotic resistance of bacteria embedded in a biofilm. *Virulence, 4*(3): 223–9. Available at: https://pubmed.ncbi.nlm.nih.gov/23380871/

Strauss, S, Glasziou, P, Richardson, W and Haynes, B (2019) *Evidence-based Medicine: How to Practice and Teach EBM* (5th edn). Edinburgh: Elsevier.

Stuttle, B (2010) Non-medical prescribing in a team context, in Courtenay, M, Taylor, C and Bailey, V (2017) Nurse prescribing: an essential requirement or an expensive luxury for school nurses? *British Journal of School Nursing, 12*: 702.

Taylor, B (2021) Culturally sensitive prescribing of common symptom management drugs. *BMJ Supportive and Palliative Care* [online]. 12 January. Available at: https://spcare.bmj.com/content/early/2021/01/12/bmjspcare-2020-002682

Taylor, C and Bailey, V (2017) Nurse prescribing: an essential requirement or an expensive luxury for school nurses? *British Journal of School Nursing, 12*: 346–52.

The Human Medicines Regulations [2012] Available at: https://www.legislation.gov.uk/uksi/2012/1916/contents/made

The King's Fund (2017) *What is Social Prescribing?* Available at: https://www.kingsfund.org.uk/publications/social-prescribing

The Misuse of Drugs Regulations 2001 (SI 2001/3998) Available at: https://www.legislation.gov.uk/uksi/2001/3998/contents/made

The Misuse of Drugs (Amendment No.2) (England, Wales and Scotland) Regulations [2012] Available at: https://www.legislation.gov.uk/uksi/2012/973/made

The Prescription Only Medicines (Human Use) Order [1997] Available at: https://www.legislation.gov.uk/uksi/1997/1830/contents

Tierney, A (1998) Nursing models: extant or extinct? *Journal of Advanced Nursing, 28*: 77–86.

UK Family Law Reform Act [1969]. Available at: https://www.legislation.gov.uk/ukpga/1969/46/contents

UK Medicines Information (UKMi) (2020) *What are the Considerations when Crushing Tablets or Opening Capsules in a Care Home Setting?* Prepared by UK Medicines Information (UKMi) pharmacists for NHS healthcare professionals. Available at: https://www.sps.nhs.uk/articles/crushing-tablets-or-opening-capsules-in-a-care-home-setting/

United Nations General Assembly, Convention on the Rights of the Child, 20 November 1989, United Nations, Treaty Series, vol. *1577*, p. 3. Available at: https://www.refworld.org/docid/3ae6b38f0.html

Vincer, K and Kaufman, G (2017) Balancing shared decision making with ethical principles in optimising medicines. *Nurse Prescribing, 15*(12): 594–9.

Wainwright, J and Canning, D (2008) Non-medical prescriber audit: evidence of CPD. *Nurse Prescribing, 6*(1): 21–5.

Weglicki, RS, Reynolds, J and Rivers, PH (2015) Continuing professional development needs of nursing and allied health professionals with responsibility for prescribing. *Nurse Education Today, 35*(1): 227–31. Available at: https://doi.org/10.1016/j.nedt.2014.08.009

West, M (2021) *The Key Components of Effective Teamworking during the COVID-19 Crisis.* Available at: https://people.nhs.uk/teamworking/the-key-components-of-effective-teamworking-during-the-covid-19-crisis/

West, M and Lyubovnikova, J (2012) Illusions of team working in health care. *Journal of Health Organization and Management* [online], *27*(1):134–42. Available at: https://onlinelibrary.wiley.com/doi/pdf/10.1111/j.1754-9434.2011.01397.x

West, M and Lyubovnikova, J (2013) Real teams or pseudo teams? The changing landscape needs a better map. *Industrial and Organizational Psychology* [online], *5*(1): 25–8. Available at: https://doi.org/10.1108/14777261311311843

While, A (2020) Life is for living: the contribution of the arts and gardens. *British Journal of Community Nursing, 25*(3).

Wikibooks (2017) *English Tort Law/Introduction* [online]. The Free Textbook Project. Available at: https://en.wikibooks.org/w/index.php?title=English_Tort_Law/Introduction&oldid=3214995

Williamson v East London & City HA [1998]. Available at: https://www.i-law.com/ilaw/doc/view.htm?id=304907

World Health Organization (WHO) (2002) *Safety of Medicines: A Guide to Detecting and Reporting Adverse Drug Reactions. Why Health Professionals Need to Take Action.* Geneva: WHO. Available at: www.who.int

World Health Organization (WHO) (2017) *Global Patient Safety Challenge 'Medication Without Harm'.* Geneva: WHO. Available at: https://www.who.int/patientsafety/medication-safety/en/

World Health Organization (WHO) (2018) *European Health Report 2018 Capturing the health 2020 core values* Available at: https://www.euro.who.int/en/data-and-evidence/european-health-report/european-health-report-2018/report-by-chapters/chapter-3-capturing-the-health-2020-core-values

World Health Organization (WHO) (2020a) *Antimicrobial Resistance Fact Sheet.* Available at: https://www.who.int/news-room/fact-sheets/detail/antibiotic-resistance

World Health Organization (WHO) (2020b) *10 Global Health Issues to Track in 2021.* Available at: https://www.who.int/news-room/spotlight/10-global-health-issues-to-track-in-2021

World Health Organization (WHO) (2020c) *Screening Programmes: A Short Guide. Increase Effectiveness, Maximize Benefits and Minimize Harm* [online]. Copenhagen, Denmark: WHO. Available at: https://www.euro.who.int/en/publications/abstracts/screening-programmes-a-short-guide.-increase-effectiveness,-maximize-benefits-and-minimize-harm-2020

World Health Organization (WHO) (2021a) *Public Health Services* [online]. Available at: https://www.euro.who.int/en/health-topics/Health-systems/public-health-services/public-health-services

World Health Organization (WHO) (2021b) *Fact Sheet: Cancer.* Available at: https://www.who.int/news-room/fact-sheets/detail/cancer

Wright, L and Jokhi, R (2020) Achieving and maintaining competency as a nurse independent non-medical prescriber. *Journal of Prescribing Practice, 2*(12): 2–7.

Xia, N and Li, H(2018) Loneliness, social isolation, and cardiovascular health. *Antioxidants and Redox Signaling, 28*(9): 837–51. Available at: https://doi.org/10.1089/ars.2017.7312

Yuwen, P, Chen, W, Lv, H, Feng, C, Li, Y, Zhang, T, Hu, P, Guo, J, Tian, Y, Liu, L, Sun, J and Zhang, Y (2017) Albumin and surgical site infection risk in orthopaedics: a meta-analysis. *BMC Surgery, 17*(1): 7. Available at: https://www.ncbi.nlm.nih.gov/pmc/articles/PMC5238522/

Index